MCQ TUTOR for students of PATHOLOGY

MCQ TUTOR
for students of
PATHOLOGY

BERNARD LENNOX
M.D., Ph.D., F.R.C.Path., F.R.C.P.(G), M.R.C.P.
*Titular professor, department of pathology at the
Western Infirmary, University of Glasgow*

WILLIAM HEINEMANN MEDICAL BOOKS LTD
LONDON

First published 1975
Reprinted 1976
Reprinted 1979

ISBN 0 433 19/50 3

Text set in 10/11 pt. IBM Century, printed and bound
in Great Britain at The Pitman Press, Bath

CONTENTS

FOREWORD

INSTRUCTIONS

Nowadays practically everyone is so familiar with M.C.Q. that detailed instructions are hardly necessary. For most of these questions, you have to choose the best answer from five given: note that it is the *best* answer, not necessarily the only possible answer, and you are expected to assume such common sense conditions as the present day and average U.K. medical situations unless otherwise indicated. While usually it is the one correct answer you are looking for, you may at times be asked contrary-wise to find the one incorrect answer among four that are correct: but the latter variety you will always find signalled by a *NOT* or similar negative word in large capitals. The cases where one-from-five questions have been grouped together to share a common answer list, though superficially different in appearance, should not cause any difficulty.

There are also some "true/false" questions, which have to be treated in a quite different way, by deciding whether each of the statements presented is T (true) or F (false). These are indicated by a "TF?" after each statement: also they are collected together into a single group within each section. (Those with experience of TF questions as usually set in this country may be uneasy at finding them numbered as separate questions, and not grouped rigidly into fives: but the conventional groups-of-five format is the result of a historical accident which need not concern us here and has no real relation to the nature of TF questions.)

Self marking

You will find it best to write down your answers on a piece of paper before turning over the page for the answer which (usually with notes) is on the *verso* side. You can if you wish then give yourself a score for each completed section. For the TF questions give yourself *one* mark for each correct answer, and subtract *one* for each incorrect: for the rest of the questions, take *two* marks for each correct, and take off a *half* mark for each incorrect. (The reasoning behind this will be found in the appendix, and there if you need it you will also find guidance on the matter of guessing or leaving alone when your answer is in doubt.)

Because of differences between different schools (not so much in standards as in content and in the precise point in the course at which examinations are held) too much reliance should not be placed on the actual figure obtained. An average Glasgow undergraduate would score in the upper sixties for most sections: the high flyers should be found in the eighties, the high risk candidates under fifty. Postgraduates aiming at examinations like the Primary F.R.C.S. (who, though this book was not written specifically for them, may find it of use) should not be satisfied with less than 90%.

Some questions have been labelled "(e)" for *easy* and/or *essential*. You should be able to answer all or nearly all of these. Of course it makes no difference to your mark on an M.C.Q. paper *which* questions you answer right, only how many. But elsewhere — in vivas, for instance — this does not apply: there are gaps in knowledge which set alarm bells ringing in the examiner's mind when he identifies them. Those included here are only a random sample of such items.

Objectives

It is hoped that in addition to self-assessment those who use this book will learn a little by the way. The questions have been less formally worded than is usual in examinations; partly because it is to be assumed that (since you have no one to outwit but yourself) it is not necessary to allow for deliberate misunderstanding: partly because it has made it easier to frame them so as to encourage thought as to why the right answers are right and (equally important) the wrong answers are wrong. If after reading the notes you find the reasons still obscure, you would be well advised to consult your books or your teachers. If you knew every fact in this book (but nothing else) you would still be altogether inadequately equipped with knowledge of pathology either for passing an examination or for your subsequent career: but if you can honestly say you understand *why* these answers are right you will at least possess a thin thread of comprehension running right through the subject.

Since Glasgow is the largest British medical school it is not unreasonable to take its course as a guide to coverage: but as the course is fairly comprehensive these chapters should be adequate for most people. Many people will find whole chapters or sections omittable, and even with the systems you have covered in class you may well find aspects unfamiliar to you. But all of it is ground you will have to cover some day, so even areas that seem superfluous to you now will not be wasted.

I have avoided any attempt to be very up-to-date, and I believe there is nothing in here that cannot be found in or deduced from a recent edition of any good student text book.

Though I take personal responsibility for all the questions in this book, any virtues they may have is the result of prolonged collaboration with and criticism by practically everyone who has been a member of the department of pathology at the Western Infirmary, Glasgow, during the last twenty years, helped by the many students who have constructively criticized our products. Among experts from whom I have learnt most are Professor J. R. Anderson, Dr. John Gordon, Dr. Terence Harris and the members of the A.S.M.E. Research and Assessment committee. I am particularly glad that my secretary, Mrs. Anne Macleod, has had this opportunity of demonstrating her skill in laying out M.C.Q. question papers.

1. INFLAMMATION AND HEALING

(e)*
1.01. Which one of the following is _NOT_ a cardinal sign of
inflammation?

    A.   Fever
    B.   Heat
    C.   Pain
    D.   Redness
    E.   Swelling.

(e)
1.02. An otherwise healthy young adult develops a haematoma
in the upper arm as a result of a blow, and this becomes
infected with staphylococci and produces a local abscess
4 cm. in diameter. Which one of the following is the
LEAST likely accompaniment?

    F.   Enlarged axillary lymph nodes
    G.   Leucopenia (fewer than 4,000 WBC per mm^3 of blood)
    H.   Local tenderness
    J.   Mild fever
    K.   Pus yellow in colour.

1.03. _NOT_ a useful effect of drainage of lymph from the site of
a small abscess:

    L.   Concentration of plasma proteins at site
    M.   Phagocytosis of micro-organisms in lymph node
    N.   Promotion of antibody formation in lymph node
    O.   Relief of tension at site
    P.   Removal of breakdown products from site.

*"(e)" stands for easy and/or essential: see Foreword p. viii.

Answers overleaf

1.01. A.

Fever is a frequent accompaniment of major inflammations, but the cardinal signs refer to local findings only.

1.02. G.

Neutrophile leucocytosis is almost certain to be present. Suppose you *did* find leucopenia in a patient with a staphylococcal abscess, what would you suspect? (See Deferred Notes.)*

1.03. L.

Since lymphatic walls have little or no filtration effect, no concentration of proteins occurs as a result of loss of fluid to the lymphatics.

*"Deferred Notes" will be found under the appropriate question number in a separate chapter, beginning on p. 139.

1.04. In acute inflammation the exudate has a higher protein content than normal tissue fluid chiefly because?

Q. Breakdown of tissue cells releases protein
R. Capillary walls are more permeable
S. Increased blood flow brings more protein into the area
T. Intracapillary pressure is raised
U. Plasma cells secrete gamma globulin.

1.05. *NOT* true of the neutrophile polymorphs in purulent inflammation caused by staphylococci?

V. Attracted to staphylococci by specific agents called staphylotaxin V, W, X, etc.
W. Die and autolyse in large numbers
X. Form the chief constituent of pus
Y. Phagocytose bacteria
Z. Serve as a source of numerous proteolytic enzymes chiefly lysosomal.

1.06. An abscess of any size can hardly ever undergo complete resolution because it?

A. Is always full of polymorph breakdown products
B. Is a form of chronic inflammation
C. Is prevented from healing by the pus it contains
D. Nearly always involves some destruction of specialized tissue
E. Nearly always requires surgical incision.

1.07. If the following events in the healing of a properly sutured surgical wound were placed in correct order, which would come *FOURTH*?

F. Fibrin clot
G. Incision
H. Inflammatory reaction
J. Laying down of collagen
K. Multiplication of fibroblasts.

Answers overleaf

1.04. R.

This (with similar changes in venules) is the key event in the production of the fluid exudate and in determining its content. Q may often contribute also in the later stages.

1.05. V.

No specific chemotactic materials have been identified: the word staphylotaxin is an invention of my own, and so far as I know however plausible it sounds no such thing exists. A question of this type is best answered by elimination, and in effect tests your confidence that all the rest are true.

1.06. D.

Destruction of specialized tissue involves healing by fibrosis, hence no resolution. An abscess in a serous cavity is a partial exception, but usually leaves adhesions.

1.07. K.

The order is probably G, H, F, K, J. The fibrin clot might result from minor oozing of blood before the inflammatory reaction produced its exudate, but this would only exchange H and F.

1.08. Rate per day of regeneration of an axon of a peripheral nerve under favourable circumstances is nearest to:

L. 100 nm.
M. 1 μm.
N. 25 μm.
O. 250 μm.
P. 3 mm.

1.09. If a postage-stamp sized skin graft of the patient's own skin is placed on an area of clean granulations in a healing wound, after about a week a thin bluish-white dry margin appears round the graft and spreads at a rate of about 1 mm. a day. What is it?

Q. Epidermis alone
R. Epidermis and dermis together
S. Dermis alone
T. Specialized inflammatory exudate
U. Dried fibrin.

1.10. Chronic inflammation is best defined as?

V. Inflammation lasting a week
W. Inflammation lasting a month
X. Inflammation lasting three months
Y. Active inflammation occurring at the same time as healing
Z. Inflammation in which lymphocytes and plasma cells predominate.

1.11—16. Generally accepted as chemical mediators of inflammation:

1.11. Aspirin T/F?*
1.12. Bradykinin T/F?
1.13. 5 HT T/F?
1.14. Lymphocyte permeability factor T/F?
1.15. Nitrosamine T/F?
1.16. Proaccelerin T/F?

*"TF?" stands for True or False?: see Foreword p. vii.

Answers overleaf

1.08. P.

This assumes growth of an axon down intact neurilemma. It is a good deal faster than most people expect.

1.09. Q.

This is the result of simple multiplication of epidermal cells. U. might form a scab, but this would look different and not spread in this way. Does this have anything to do with the contraction of scars? (See Deferred Notes.)

1.10. Y.

This is an agreed definition with which it is unwise to argue. A cystitis may last for years, and so long as no ulceration or scarring of the bladder occurs, it is still technically not chronic inflammation. Many chronic inflammations — e.g. osteitis and actinomycosis — produce polymorphs indefinitely. (Not all pathologists agree with this: make sure you know the local views).

1.12., 1.13., 1.14. T., rest F.

Aspirin *reduces* exudate formation after the early histamine-like phase. Nitrosamine is a carcinogen and proaccelerin a clotting factor.

1.17—22. Macrophages:

    1.17. Are capable of multiplication T/F?
    1.18. Are essentially the same cell type as the blood
           monocytes T/F?
    1.19. Ditto for the Kupffer cells of the liver T/F?   ?
    1.20. Live longer than polymorphs T/F?
    1.21. Play an essential role in organization of fibrin T/F?
    1.22. Split red cells but not haemoglobin T/F?

1.23—27. Complete restoration to normal usually occurs in an adult after:

    1.23. Necrosis of peripheral half of every lobule of the
           liver T/F?
    1.24. Ditto for central half T/F?
    1.25. Fracture of clavicle T/F?
    1.26. Transection of a voluntary muscle T/F?
    1.27. Transection of a tendon T/F?

Answers overleaf

1.17. T., 1.18., 1.19. T.

These are all reticuloendothelial cells with similar functions.

1.20. T.

The polymorph is a post-mitotic cell that rarely lives longer than 4 days, the macrophage is capable of indefinite survival and of multiplication.

1.21. T.

Endothelial cells, fibroblasts, macrophages are the essential three.

1.22. F.

Hb is split into iron, haem, and globin in the macrophage.

1.23., 1.24. T.

Near-complete necrosis of the epithelium of the lobule is needed to prevent regeneration so long as the reticulin framework is intact. (This is perhaps not so certainly true for peripheral necrosis as for central.)

1.25. T.

Reconstruction of the callus ultimately leads to disappearance of all trace of the fracture.

1.26., 1.27. F.

Scars are left in both cases. The collagen of a tendon is too specialized to be perfectly regenerated.

1.28—32. Common complications of healing of an abdominal laparotomy wound:

    1.28. Post-operative wound infection with *Streptococcus faecalis* T/F?

    1.29. Incisional hernia T/F?

    1.30. Bone formation in scar T/F?

    1.31. Intestinal obstruction due to contraction of scar T/F?

    1.32. Tumour formation T/F?

Answers overleaf

1.28. F.

This is rarely a pathogen.

1.29. T.

Due to stretching of scar.

1.30. T.

Metaplasia in old hyaline abdominal scars is not unusual, though perhaps not really common.

1.31. F.

Intestinal obstruction may result from adhesions, but not from change in the scar itself.

1.32. F.

Very rare at this site. Scar cancers arise mostly in wounds kept open by sinuses or ulcers, or sometimes in scars exposed to prolonged sunlight.

2. SPECIAL INFECTIONS AND IMMUNOPATHOLOGY

2.01. Sensitivity to the tubercle bacillus depends on the presence of the appropriate type of:

A. α-globulin
B. β-globulin
C. B-lymphocytes
D. T-lymphocytes
E. Reagins.

2.02. The best histological evidence of resistance to the tubercle bacillus is the number or amount of?

F. Caseation
G. Collagen
H. Epithelioid cells
J. Giant cells
K. Lymphocytes

2.03. Discharge of tubercle bacilli in large numbers into the thoracic duct would most probably produce?

L. Caseation of glands of neck
M. Caseation of glands of upper mediastinum
N. Generalized miliary tuberculosis
O. Miliary tuberculosis of the lungs especially
P. Pleural effusion.

2.04. The chief cause of death in young children with primary tuberculosis is:

Q. Bronchopneumonia
R. Lymph spread
S. Meningitis
T. Miliary spread
U. Renal involvement.

Answers overleaf

2.01. D.

The thymic lymphocytes of cell-bound immunity.

2.02. G.

Successful encapsulation of the tubercle is good evidence of resistance.

2.03. O.

The pathway is thoracic duct to great veins to right heart to lungs: hence miliary tuberculosis, with the lungs being first affected.

2.04. S.

Tuberculous meningitis was the great killer when primary tuberculosis was common.

2.05. A man who denies venereal exposure has an ulcer on his foreskin of a few weeks' duration. Biopsy of the edge of the ulcer suggests syphilis. Which test would be of most help in confirming this?

V. Blood culture
W. Dark ground examination of exudate from ulcer.
X. Kahn test
Y. Skin test using treponemal antigen
Z. Wasserman reaction.

2.06. John Hunter inoculated himself with syphilitic material and, so it is said, in consequence died suddenly many years later. His cause of death in this case was probably?

A. General paralysis of the insane
B. Gumma of liver
C. Myocardial infarct
D. Pulmonary embolism
E. Rupture of aortic aneurysm.

2.07. The less destructive of the two main forms of leprosy affects especially?

F. Liver
G. Lymph nodes
H. Nose
J. Oesophagus
K. Peripheral nerves.

2.08. Characteristic of pus seen in actinomycosis?

L. Contains small firm yellow bodies
M. Foul smelling
N. Green
O. Pinkish and translucent
P. Thin and blood-tinged.

Answers overleaf

2.05. W.

The best test for primary syphilis, which is the probable stage here. X and Z become positive later. V and Y are not relevant to syphilis.

2.06. E.

C and D cause sudden death but are not related to syphilis, A and B are syphilitic but do not cause sudden death.

2.07. K.

This is "tuberculoid" or "neural" type (with tuberculosis-type cell-mediated immune reaction). The other type, with the familiar lesions of face and nose, is "lepromatous".

2.08. L.

"Sulphur granules", which are colonies. What might the others be? (See Deferred Notes.)

2.09. The common childhood infection of mouth and throat called thrush is due to?

Q. *Candida albicans*
R. *Plasmodium vivax*
S. *Sarcoptes scabiei*
T. *Taenia echinococcus*
U. *Toxoplasma gondii.*

2.10—13. Plasma cells are:

      2.10. Basophilic because they are packed with mito-chondria T/F?
(e) 2.11. Derived from B lymphocytes T/F?
(e) 2.12. Principal source of IgG T/F?
      2.13. Usually present in the exudate of a five-day old acute inflammatory focus T/F?

2.14—18. Auto-immune diseases:

(e) 2.14. Asthma T/F?
      2.15. Atrophic gastritis in pernicious anaemia T/F?
(e) 2.16. Hashimoto's disease T/F?
      2.17. Histoplasmosis T/F?
      2.18. Sympathetic ophthalmia T/F?

2.19. At the site of an Arthus reaction produced by the last of a long course of injections of a soluble antigen, which one of the following would one *NOT* expect to find at the site?

V. Antigen
W. Complement
X. Immunoglobulin
Y. Polymorphs
Z. Transformed lymphocytes.

Answers overleaf

2.09. Q.

It is a fungus, usually a saprophyte, sometimes causing superficial infection as thrush, occasionally more serious disseminated opportunistic disease.

Do you know (a) what "opportunistic" means here and (b) what the other organisms (all common) are? (See Deferred Notes.)

2.10. F.

The basophilia is due to the RNA in ribosomes, involved in manufacture of γ-globulin. Excess of mitochondria makes cytoplasm eosinophilic.

2.11. T., 2.12. T.

2.13. F.

Not usually seen till local antibody response becomes important.

2.14. F.

2.15. T.

Autoantibodies against oxyntic cells are usually found.

2.16. T. The classical example (thyroid).

2.17. F. A fungus infection (lung).

2.18. T.

The first recognized example of autoimmunity (eye).

2.19. Z.

This is a reaction to complement-containing antigen-antibody complexes, and cell-mediated responses are not concerned.

2.20. A mouse of pure strain X has been made tolerant by an injection of Y strain cells at birth, and now as an adult bears a skin graft of strain Y. It can be induced to reject this graft by?

    A. Freund's adjuvant repeatedly injected.
    B. Lymphocytes of strain X
    C. Lymphocytes of strain Y
    D. Lymphocytes of a third unrelated strain
    E. X-rays in high dosage.

2.21—24. Identify the four main types of allergy — i.e. the four main ways in which immune reactions cause disease.

2.21. Type I	F.	Anaphylactic
2.22. Type II	G.	Arthus
2.23. Type III	H.	Cell-mediated
2.24. Type IV	J.	Cytotoxic
	K.	Immune-complex.

2.25—30. Having made sure from the last question group that you know the types of allergy, what are the types of the following diseases? (You may have to use answers more than once.)

2.25. Asthma	L.	Type I
2.26. Farmer's lung	M.	Type II
2.27. Hashimoto's disease	N.	Type III
2.28. Rhesus disease	O.	Type IV
2.29. Fever, rash and joint swelling a week after tetanus antiserum injection	P.	None of these.
2.30. Sudden death shortly after the same		

Answers overleaf

2.20. B.

Lymphocytes from a normal X strain mouse will survive in our mouse, but will recognize the graft as foreign.

2.21. F.

IgE, reagin, reacts to release histamine from basophiles: e.g. hay-fever.

2.22. J.

Direct cell damage by antibodies: e.g. blood group iso-antibodies.

2.23. K.

Damage chiefly by complement held by the antibody-antigen reaction (e.g. Arthus, glomerulonephritis).

2.24. H.

(Or delayed type). Damage by sensitized lymphocytes, e.g. tuberculin.
(G. Arthus, is merely a subgroup of Type III.)

2.25. and 2.30. L.

Anaphylactic, the second being classical anaphylaxis.

2.26. N.

Of Arthus type, with excess of antibody and local precipitation of the complex.

2.27. and 2.28. M.

Both direct cell damage by antibodies. IV is probably also involved in Hashimoto.

2.29. N.

This is serum sickness, with soluble circulating complex produced by excess of antigen.

3. TUMOURS

3.01—3. Definitions?

  (e) 3.01. Benign epithelial tumour   A.   Adenoma
          of gland-like structure   B.   Carcinoma
  (e) 3.02. Benign epithelial tumour   C.   Cystadenoma
          with dilated glandular   D.   Papilloma
          spaces   E.   Sarcoma.
  (e) 3.03. Malignant tumour of
          connective tissue

3.04. The most fundamental difference between a tumour and a normal tissue is that it?

  F.   Forms a lump
  G.   Grows faster
  H.   Has more mitoses
  J.   Keeps on growing when not required for needs of the body
  K.   Tends to ulcerate easily.

(e) 3.05. In examining a biopsy of a primary tumour, the *clearest* evidence of malignancy is provided by?

  L.   Absence of capsule
  M.   Basophilia of cytoplasm
  N.   Invasion of surrounding structures
  O.   Excess of mitoses
  P.   Nuclear aberrations.

Answers overleaf

3.01. A.

3.02. C.

3.03. E.

3.04. J.

All of these are true of most tumours, but all the rest can be true of normal tissues (e.g. F of a fracture callus).

3.05. N.

All these features are usually seen in malignant tumours but invasion is (apart from metastases, not to be seen in a biopsy of the primary) the most certain indication.

3.06. The large size and deep basophilia of the nuclei of tumour cells is due to?

Q. Accumulation of mucopolysaccharides
R. Fusion of nuclei
S. Increase of transfer RNA
T. Increased number of chromosomes
U. Increased size of chromosomes.

3.07—9. Mode of spread in each of these examples of metastasis of carcinoma?

(e) 3.07. Gastric carcinoma to anterior free surface of rectum
     3.08. Prostatic carcinoma to lumbar vertebral bodies
(e) 3.09. Rectal carcinoma to liver

V. Blood spread (portal)
W. Blood spread (systemic)
X. Lymph spread
Y. Transperitoneal
Z. Retrograde venous.

3.10. A biopsy of a small lump above the left clavicle in a man of 60 shows metastatic tumour in a lymph node. Without knowing the precise histology of the tumour, which of the following would you regard as the most probable primary?

A. Adenocarcinoma of tail of pancreas
B. Malignant astrocytoma of left temporal lobe
C. Osteosarcoma of left humerus
D. Rodent ulcer of chin
E. Wilms' tumour of kidney.

3.11. Of common tumours, the one in which inappropriate enzyme secretion is recognized most often is the?

F. Clear-cell of kidney
G. Oat-cell of bronchus
H. Osteosarcoma
J. Scirrhous of breast
K. Scirrhous of stomach.

Answers overleaf

3.06. T.

Most malignant tumour cells have more than the normal number of chromosomes, which is sometimes many times multiplied.

3.07. Y.

The recto-vesical (or recto-uterine) pouch is a common site of lodgement of cancer cells within the peritoneum. What curious example of the same process involves the ovary? (See Deferred Notes.)

3.08. Z.

Due to anomalous tidal flow in vertebral veins resulting from differences in pressure above and below diaphragm: hence blood sometimes flows directly from the prostatic venous flexus into the lower lumbar vertebrae. Does this apply anywhere else? (See Deferred Notes.)

3.09. V.

3.10. A.

Widespread lymphatic metastasis is particularly characteristic of pancreatic carcinomas. Rodents (D) and intra-cranial tumours (B) do not in general metastasize: sarcomas (C) in general do not spread by lymphatics: and Wilms' tumour (E) is almost confined to childhood.

3.11. G.

Fairly common if looked for: chiefly 5HT, ACTH and para-thormone. None of the others has any special tendency in this direction. What *appropriate* hormone do renal carcinomas some-times secrete? (See Deferred Notes.)

3.12. Teratomas arise chiefly in?

    L. Gonads
    M. Heart
    N. Liver
    O. Mediastinum
    P. Sacrum.

3.13. The most striking example of a cancer which is relatively rare in this country but very common in most of the undeveloped and tropical countries is:

    Q. Breast
    R. Bronchus
    S. Colon
    T. Liver
    U. Stomach.

3.14—16. These observations best fit which theory of the origin of cancer?

3.14. A course of croton oil painting increase incidence of skin tumours if given after methylcholanthrene, but not before

3.15. The incidence of most common tumours of man is roughly proportional to the 7th power of the age

(e) 3.16. The Shope papilloma can be transmitted by a cell-free filtrate of the tumour.

    V. Carcinogen/cocarcinogen (two stage) theory
    W. Contact inhibition theory
    X. Immunological surveillance theory
    Y. Multiple mutation theory
    Z. Virus theory.

Answers overleaf

3.12. L.

Malignant testicular in the male, benign ovarian ('dermoid cysts') in the female. They are rarely seen elsewhere, though a few are seen in O and there is an infantile form seen chiefly in P.

3.13. T.

One of the commonest cancers in most of the tropics. R has the reverse trend, and so have Q and S to a milder degree. U is common nearly everywhere, but we have a relatively lower incidence than most western countries.

3.14. V.

A cocarcinogen will act after induction of the essential change by the carcinogen.

3.15. Y.

If it took about 6 mutations, occurring independently at random, to produce a cancer, the fact would be explained.

3.16. Z.

The filtrate does in fact contain a virus. And so at least *that* tumour is virus produced. (Note that these five 'theories' are not mutually exclusive: they may well all be aspects of the truth about cancer, or at least some cancers.)

3.17—21. Well-established causes of cancer in man:

    3.17. Asbestos and bronchial carcinoma T/F?
    3.18. Burkitt's tumour (African lymphoma) and the EB virus T/F?
    3.19. Deep X-rays and chronic myeloid leukaemia T/F?
    3.20. Food preservatives and cancer of the stomach T/F?
    3.21. Sunlight and rodent ulcer T/F?

3.22—26. Well-established examples of chemical carcinogenesis in man:

    3.22. Aniline dyes (β-naphthylamine) and bladder cancer T/F?
    3.23. Arsenic and skin cancer T/F?
    3.24. Cigarette smoke and colonic cancer T/F?
    3.25. Radio-iodine and thyroid cancer T/F?
    3.26. Soot and cancer of the scrotum T/F?

Answers overleaf

3.17. T.

Both bronchial carcinoma and mesothelioma.

3.18. T.

The nature of the association with EB virus is uncertain however, and some would answer otherwise.

3.19. T.

3.20. F.

The cause of gastric cancer is in general unknown.

3.21. T.

Mostly in the fair-skinned in sunny climates.

3.22. T.

Remember the crucial conversion to the hydroxy form.

3.23. T.

This applies both to those who take arsenic for long periods medicinally, and to workers with powdered arsenic.

3.24. F.

Cigarettes produce cancer of air passage and (probably) the bladder.

3.25. F.

Not *chemical* carcinogenesis: but in any event (perhaps because of care in its use) cases in man are negligible.

3.26. T.

The first industrial cancer identified (Percival Pott, 1775).

4. MISCELLANEOUS GENERAL PATHOLOGY

4.01. For a tissue to be necrotic, it must not only be dead but also?

    A. Be pale to the naked eye
    B. Be sterile
    C. Form part of a living body
    D. Have undergone autolysis
    E. Involve part of a solid organ.

4.02. Mostly closely concerned with autolysis?

    F. Centriole
    G. Coarse endoplasmic reticulum
    H. Golgi apparatus
    J. Lysosome
    K. Nuclear membrane.

4.03. Rapid liquefaction of necrotic areas is especially characteristic of?

    L. Brain
    M. Heart
    N. Kidney
    O. Liver
    P. Spleen.

(e) 4.04. Gangrene is necrosis plus?

    Q. Dessication
    R. Infection
    S. Involvement of a limb
    T. Involvement of skin
    U. Putrefaction.

Answers overleaf

4.01. C.

Meat on a butcher's slab is dead but not necrotic.

4.02. J.

Release of proteolytic enzymes from the lysosome is a major factor in breakdown of the cell proteins after death of the cell.

4.03. L.

This is "colliquative necrosis". The rapid softening of large areas of the brain is very characteristic of the infarcts of cerebral thrombosis. Factors include the presence of myelin, which becomes fluid when released, and smallness of content of the relatively resistant collagen.

4.04. U.

"If it doesn't smell it's not gangrene."

(e) **4.05. Gas gangrene is necrosis produced by?**

    V.   Extensive muscle damage
    W. Infection with Clostridia
    X.   Infection with Pyocyaneus
    Y.   Surgical emphysema
    Z.   Traumatic damage to arteries.

4.06. _NOT_ producing a marked increase of fat in the liver?

    A. Carbon tetrachloride poisoning
    B. Chronic alcoholism
    C. Extreme obesity
    D. Severe pernicious anaemia
    E. Threonine deficiency.

4.07. _NOT_ a characteristic site of deposition of calcium salts?

    F. Atheromatous patches in aorta
    G. Healed caseous tuberculous lesion
    H. Old midline laparotomy wound
    J. Pyramids of kidney
    K. Wall of inferior vena cava.

4.08–10. Connected with the origin of these brown pigments?

(e)   4.08. Haemosiderin   L.   Benzidine poisoning
          4.09. Lipofuscin   M. Breakdown of red blood cells
          4.10. Melanin   N.   DOPA
                            O.   Old age
                            P.   Sludging of blood.

Answers overleaf

4.05. W.

Infection with the anaerobic gas-producing Clostridia (chiefly *welchii*, *oedematiens* and *septicum*) is essential, though factors such as V and Z may encourage the infection.

4.06. E.

Methionine is the only amino-acid deficiency which is associated with fatty change in the liver.

4.07. K.

The common factor in the rest is probably low CO_2 content or high pH. Veins are usually well supplied with CO_2.

4.08. M.

The iron of haem combines with apoferritin to form ferritin, from which granules of haemosiderin are derived.

4.09. O.

Accumulates with age especially in heart and liver.

4.10. N.

The characteristic intermediate in the oxidation of tyrosine before it polymerizes to form melanin.

4.11. The deleterious effects of a single exposure to irradiation appear at very different times after the event. If the following were placed in order of the time of most probable occurrence in a population which would be *FOURTH?*

Q. Death of descendant from gene defect
R. Extensive ulceration of gut
S. Leukaemia
T. Massive haemorrhage
U. Massive infection.

4.12—14. Who discovered or invented?

4.12. "All cells come from another cell", infarcts and leukaemia

4.13. A kind of anaemia and an endocrine disease

4.14. A kind of cirrhosis, the stethoscope, and the unity of tuberculosis.

V. Giovanni Morgagni
W. René Laennec
X. Thomas Addison
Y. Rudolf Virchow
Z. Ludwig Aschoff.

4.15—17. Cause of atrophy of these tissues?

4.15. Bone, producing local depressions on surface

4.16. Liver, diffuse, with reduction in size of cells

4.17. Thyroid epithelium in Hashimoto's disease.

A. Autoimmunity
B. Low level of pituitaryhormone
C. Pressure
D. Starvation
E. Vitamin deficiency.

Answers overleaf

4.11. S.

The order would be:— R (direct damage), about 10 days: T (platelet loss) and U (polymorph loss) both 2—6 weeks: S, 5 years + : Q, indefinite. The dose required is in inverse order, from 500r for R to minute for Q.

4.12. Y.

'Omnia cellula e cellule' is one of the key propositions of biology as well as pathology.

4.13. X.

Pernicious anaemia and adrenal deficiency.

4.14. W.

Laennec's cirrhosis is an old name for the macronodular type. He recognized tuberculosis as a single disease, characterized by tubercles, about fifty years before the discovery of the bacillus. Who were the other two? (See Deferred Notes.)

4.15. C.

Pressure on the surface of the bone produces local osteoclastic resorption.

4.16. D.

Seen in any severe malnutrition — e.g. many cancer deaths.

4.17. A.

TSH will be raised, if affected at all.

4.18—24. Enlargement (hyperplasia or hypertrophy) results from the demand for increased functional activity in:

4.18. Left ventricle in mitral stenosis T/F?
4.19. Opposite kidney after nephrectomy T/F?
4.20. Opposite testis after orchidectomy T/F?
4.21. Prostrate in urethral obstruction T/F?
4.22. Right ventricle in superior vena cava obstruction T/F?
4.23. Sciatic nerve in marathon runners T/F?
4.24. Thyroid after treatment with antithyroid drugs T/F?

Answers overleaf

4.18. F.

(See 4.22.)

4.19. T.

By enlargement of nephrons, no new ones being formed.

4.20. F.

Leydig cells compensate, but not the tubules, and the effect of the Leydig cells on total size is negligible.

4.21. F.

Prostatic enlargement causes (or produces the effect of) urethral obstruction, not the other way round.

4.22. F.

Both here and in 4.18, since the heart is not a vacuum pump, an obstruction upstream of it cannot be compensated for by extra work by the chamber concerned.

4.23. F.

Nerve activity does not affect the size of nerves.

4.24. T.

These drugs suppress thyroid hormone production, pituitary feed-back leads to TSH increase and increase of size of thyroid.

4.25—29. Imply presence of necrosis:

(e) **4.25.** Caseation T/F?
(e) **4.26.** Cloudy swelling T/F?
    4.27. Gumma T/F?
(e) **4.28.** Infarct of kidney T/F?
    4.29. Inflammatory exudate T/F?

4.30—35. True of amyloidosis?

    4.30. Common complication of chronic tuberculosis T/F?
    4.31. Plasma gamma globulin usually raised T/F?
    4.32. Primary form usually most severe in liver, T/F?
    4.33. Secondary form involves especially spleen, liver and kidneys T/F?
    4.34. Secondary form's earliest deposits are seen round arterioles T/F?
    4.35. When fatal, most often this is due to cerebral deposits T/F?

Answers overleaf

4.25. T.

4.26. F.

Cloudy swelling is a minor reversible change.

4.27. and 4.28. T.

4.29. F.

Though many inflammatory episodes involve necrosis, it is by no means necessary — e.g. a nasal catarrh.

4.30. T.

4.31. T.

Part of the evidence that immune mechanisms are involved in some way.

4.32. F.

Very variable, but usually not liver.

4.33. T.

4.34. T.

Important in gum and rectal biopsies used for diagnosis.

4.35. F.

Renal failure chief killer, and cerebral involvement practically unknown.

5. CARDIOVASCULAR SYSTEM

(e) 5.01. If a small embolus leaves a calf vein, in which of the following is it most likely to lodge?

A. Coronary artery
B. Middle cerebral artery
C. Pulmonary artery branch
D. Renal artery branch
E. Splenic artery.

(e) 5.02. A man of 50 dies of cerebral softening after lodgement in a carotid artery of an embolus that is known to have come from a leg vein. What would you expect to find at post mortem to explain this anomalous finding?

F. Coarctation of the aorta
G. Hole in the heart (either interatrial or interventricular)
H. Portocaval anastomosis (i.e. portal vein to vena cava)
J. Recent aortic graft
K. Transposition of great vessels.

(e) 5.03. Blockage of which of these arteries is _LEAST_ likely to cause death?

L. Middle cerebral
M. Pulmonary (trunk)
N. Right coronary
O. Splenic
P. Superior mesenteric.

Answers overleaf

5.01. C.

If you got this one wrong, the anatomy examiners have been too kind to you. But see next question.

5.02. G.

This is "paradoxical embolism". The embolus has to pass through the hole from right to left. Without a shunt of this kind, such an embolus can *only* lodge in the lungs. 'K' of course is an alternative explanation, but is not compatible with survival to 50.

5.03. O.

Even total infarction of the spleen will cause only local trouble. Be sure you know what each of the others cause. (See Deferred Notes.)

5.04 —6. Rupture of aneurysms produces haemorrhage into?

	5.04. Atheromatous aneurysm	Q.	Cerebrospinal fluid
(e)	**5.05.** Berry aneurysm	R.	Duodenum
	5.06. Dissecting aneurysm	S.	Pericardium
		T.	Peritoneum
		U.	Tissues of neck.

5.07. If at post mortem you find the following, which one would make you most confident that the patient did *NOT* have systemic hypertension during life?

V. Absence of left ventricular hypertrophy
W. Histologically normal retina
X. Minimal aortic atheroma
Y. Normal adrenals
Z. Normal kidneys.

5.08. *FOURTH* in the following chain of events?

A. Hypertrophy of left ventricle
B. Pressure on renal artery
C. Rise in blood angiotensin
D. Rise in blood pressure
E. Rise in blood renin.

5.09. *FOURTH* in the following chain of events?

F. Coronary thrombosis
G. Death
H. Myocardial infarct with softening
J. Rupture of heart
K. Pressure on roots of venae cavae.

Answers overleaf

5.04. T.

Rupture of such aneurysms of the abdominal aorta into the peritoneum (or retroperitoneally) is now fairly common.

5.05. Q.

Circle of Willis and adjoining arteries.

5.06. S.

When a dissecting aneurysm ruptures, it does so most often at the aortic ring, where it is inside the pericardium.

5.07. V.

All the other organs have some association with hypertension, but V is simplest and most reliable.

5.08. D.

The simple physiological sequence is B, E, C, D, A.

5.09. K.

The order is F, H, J, K, G. J results in haemopericardium, and the immediate effect of this is to block inflow of blood into the heart at its point of lowest internal pressure (K) producing death.

(e) 5.10. The commonest cause of sudden death in the U.K. at present is?

L. Accident
M. Cerebral haemorrhage
N. Cerebral thrombosis
O. Myocardial infarction
P. Peritonitis.

5.11. If a patient who dies a week after his first attack of coronary coronary thrombosis is known to have had heart block during that week, you would expect at post mortem to find the infarct involving?

Q. Anterior wall of L.V.
R. Apex of heart
S. Left margin of L.V.
T. Upper posterior part of L.V. wall
U. Upper third of I.V. septum.

5.12. Surprisingly *RARE*?

V. Calcification of aortic valve
W. Emboli in coronary arteries
X. Fibrosis of myocardium
Y. Non-significant patency of foramen ovale
Z. Thrombus in right auricular appendage.

(e) 5.13. *NOT* a cause of left ventricular hypertrophy?

A. Aortic incompetence
B. Aortic stenosis
C. Coarctation of aorta
D. Pulmonary hypertension
E. Systemic hypertension.

Answers overleaf

5.10. O.

Could you specify a subset of the U.K. population for whom L is true? (See Deferred Notes.)

5.11. U.

Only this will interrupt the I.V. bundle near its origin.

5.12. W.

Practically never — presumably related to their peculiar origin behind the aortic cusps and the jet effect of the outflow, but the precise reason is unexplained.

5.13. D.

5.14. Heart failure in malnutrition is most probably due to:

   F.   Low blood calcium
   G. Protein lack
   H. Thiamine (vit. B) deficiency
   J.   Vit. C deficiency
   K. Vit. D deficiency.

(e) 5.15. *FOURTH* in the following chain of events?

   L.   Acute inflammation of mitral valve (pin-head vegetations)
   M. Acute rheumatic fever
   N. Death from heart failure
   O. Infarct of spleen
   P.   Mitral stenosis.

(e) 5.16. Most valuable laboratory finding in diagnosis of sub-acute bacterial endocarditis?

   Q. Evidence of haemolytic anaemia.
   R. Finding of *Strept. viridans* in blood culture
   S.   High titre of antistreptolysins
   T.   Persistent leucocytosis
   U. Red cells in urine.

5.17.—23. Accepted positive associations with increased liability to atheroma?

       5.17. Abnormally strenuous exercise in youth T/F?
(e)   5.18. Diabetes mellitus T/F?
(e)   5.19. Hypercholesterolaemia T/F?
(e)   5.20. Hypertension T/F?
       5.21. Obesity T/F?
       5.22. Persistent high blood oestrogen T/F?
       5.23. Western civilization T/F?

Answers overleaf

5.14. H.

This is cardiac beri-beri.

5.15. O.

The order should be M, L, P, O, N. If the vegetations had been large, what would the order be? (See Deferred Notes.) The infarct of the spleen of course is not the actual cause of death, merely an incident between the appearance of mitral stenosis and ultimate death.

5.16. R.

Q and U at least will usually also be positive, but less specific as evidence.

5.17. F.

5.18. T.

Probably because diabetes causes 5.19.

5.19., 20., 21. T.

Classical associations.

5.22. F.

The lower incidence in women has been ascribed to oestrogens, though treatment of males with oestrogen has had little effect.

5.23. T.

5.24 —28. Complications of severe atheroma of aorta?

    5.24. Calcification of aortic wall T/F?
    5.25. Fusiform aneurysm of ascending aorta T/F?
    5.26. Gangrene of both legs T/F?
    5.27. Infarction of ribs T/F?
    5.28. Saccular aneurysm of arch T/F?

5.29—33. A boy of twelve has a congenital 'hole-in-the-heart' 10 mm. in diameter giving free communication between left and right ventricle; he has some limitation of exercise but is not in heart failure. There is no other congenital defect. One would expect him to have:

    5.29. Hypertrophy of right ventricle T/F?
    5.30. An abnormally thick wall to the pulmonary artery T/F?
    5.31. Flow of blood in the defect predominantly from right to left T/F?
    5.32. Absence of cyanosis T/F?
    5.33. A risk of developing sub-acute bacterial endocarditis T/F?

Answers overleaf

5.24. T.

5.25. F.

While atheromatous aneurysms *can* occur anywhere in the aorta, aortic atheroma usually increases from above downward and so aneurysms are only common below the diaphragm.

5.26. T.

Result of severe atheroma at the bifurcation, producing saddle thrombus.

5.27. F.

Abundant anastomoses between intercostals prevent this.

5.28. F.

Characteristic type of syphilis.

5.29. T.

5.30. T.

5.31. F.   Work these out.
                  (See Deferred Notes.)

5.32. T.

5.33. T.

6. RESPIRATORY SYSTEM

6.01. When one has a cold and blows one's nose, the material that one blows out is?

    A.   Inflammatory exudate
    B.   Lymph
    C.   Mixture of mucus and inflammatory exudate
    D.   Mucus
    E.   Nasal gland secretions.

6.02. _NOT_ a cause of loss of ventilation capacity of the lungs?

    F.   Extensive fibrosis of lungs
    G.   Gross obesity
    H.   Obliteration of pleural cavities
    J.   Paralysis of whole diaphragm
    K.   Severe kyphoscoliosis.

6.03. _NOT_ a cause of right ventricular hypertrophy?

    L.   Extensive fibrosis of lungs
    M.   Gross obesity
    N.   Obliteration of pleural cavities
    O.   Paralysis of whole diaphragm
    P.   Severe kyphoscoliosis.

6.04. The most reliable index at post mortem of the presence of chronic bronchitis during life is?

    Q.   Atheroma of pulmonary arteries
    R.   Enlargement of bronchial mucus glands
    S.   Enlargement of hilar lymph glands
    T.   Peribronchial emphysema
    U.   Peribronchial fibrosis.

Answers overleaf

6.01. C.

This is a typical catarrhal inflammation, with outpouring of inflammatory exudate through a slightly damaged epithelium: but the nasal glands also contribute much mucus.

6.02. H.

Unless accompanied by very dense fibrosis, this has surprisingly little effect. The rest affect ventilation principally, though not solely, by limiting the range of expansion of the lungs.

6.03. N.

(See 6.02.) To emphasize that anything that interferes with lung ventilation causes R.V. hypertrophy (cor pulmonale).

6.04. R.

This correlates with the clinical definition which relies on excessive sputum production. Right ventricular hypertrophy is a useful index of the severity of disability produced by the bronchitis.

6.05. <u>NOT</u> a characteristic of lobar pneumonia?

    V.   Alveoli filled with a clotted inflammatory exudate
    W. Caused by *Strept. pneumoniae*
    X.   Good ventilation of affected lobe
    Y.   Occasionally followed by patchy residual fibrosis
    Z.   Usually undergoes rapid resolution after about a week.

(e) 6.06 The characteristic picture of *primary* tuberculosis in the lung of a child consists of?

    A.   Calcified Ghon focus
    B.   Hilar lymph node lesion
    C.   Miliary tubercles
    D.   Small focus at periphery of lung
    E.   Small focus (as D) plus lymph node lesion.

(e) 6.07. The characteristic picture of chronic lung tuberculosis in an adult with positive sputum is:

    F.   Bronchopneumonic lesion at base
    G.   Caseous lesion in hilar lymph node
    H.   Cavity at the apex
    J.   Diffuse fibrosis
    K.   Pleural effusion.

6.08. <u>NOT</u> true of the results of exposure to asbestos?

    L.   Crocidolite the most dangerous form
    M. Raised incidence of bronchial carcinoma
    N.   Raised incidence of mesothelioma
    O.   Rapid development of lung fibrosis with heavy exposure.
    P.   Triangular asbestos bodies can be found in the lungs.

Answers overleaf

6.05. X.

How can a solid lobe with its alveoli full of clotted exudate be well ventilated?

6.06. E.

This is the characteristic primary tuberculous complex.

6.07. H.

The classic lesion of adult tuberculosis. All the rest are characteristic of some other forms of the disease: what? (See Deferred Notes.)

6.08. P.

Asbestos bodies are shaped like a string of beads strung on a straight needle, not triangular.

6.09. The characteristic lung lesion of silicosis is:

    Q. Bronchiectasis
    R. Diffuse fibrosis
    S. Focal (centrilobular) emphysema
    T. Large round fibrous nodules with collagen necrosis
    U. Small round hyaline fibrous nodules

(e) 6.10. Most nearly true of the incidence of cancer of the bronchus in non-smokers in the U.K.?

    V. Nil
    W. About 1/1000 that of smokers
    X. About 1/8 that of smokers
    Y. Equal to that of smokers
    Z. In women only, equal to that of smokers.

(e) 6.11. *FOURTH* in this sequence?

    A. Bronchopneumonia of one segment of lung
    B. Carcinoma of bronchus
    C. Heavy cigarette smoking
    D. Obstruction of bronchus
    E. Squamous metaplasia of bronchial epithelium.

6.12. The essential lesion produced by the influenza virus is?

    F. Acute inflammation of smaller bronchi in apical segments
    G. Bronchopneumonia
    H. Depleted secretion of bronchial glands
    J. Necrosis of respiratory epithelium of trachea and bronchi
    K. Viral septicaemia.

Answers overleaf

6.09. U.

R could be caused (among other things) by asbestos and S by coal dust. T suggests Caplan's syndrome, seen in coal miners who also have rheumatoid arthritis.

6.10. X.

There is a large difference in both sexes, but there are some cases due to other carcinogens, and a fair number (mostly adenocarcinomas) in which no recognized carcinogen is involved.

6.11. D.

The sequence is C, E, B, D, A.

6.12. J.

This is the specific virus effect. Bronchopneumonia is a common complication due to secondary bacterial infection.

6.13—19. A pharyngeal infection with β-haemolytic streptococci may be the cause of:

(e)   6.13. Acute glomerulonephritis T/F?
      6.14. Acute rheumatic fever T/F?
      6.15. Diphtheria T/F?
(e)   6.16. Scarlet fever T/F?
(e)   6.17. Swollen tender neck glands T/F?
      6.18. Thrush T/F?
      6.19. Wound infection T/F?

Answers overleaf

6.13. T.

(Type 12: antigen-antibody complex.)

6.14. T.

(Multiple types.)

6.15. F.

Due to *Corynebacterium diphtheriae.* (So rare, as a result of immunization, that you will probably never see a case, but examiners know all about it.)

6.16. T.

(Erythogenic toxin.)

6.17. T.

Common in almost any pharyngeal infection unless very mild.

6.18. F.

Due to *Candida albicans.*

6.19. T.

E.g. if the surgeon is a carrier.

6.20—24. A major risk of lung infection results from:

      6.20. Damage to cilia of trachea and bronchi T/F?
      6.21. Heart failure T/F?
(e)   **6.22.** Loss of cough reflex T/F?
(e)   **6.23.** Obstruction of bronchus T/F?
      6.24. Pharyngitis T/F?

6.25—29. *NOT* capable of causing dust disease of the lung:

(e)   **6.25.** Asbestos T/F?
      6.26. Beryllium T/F?
(e)   **6.27.** Coal T/F?
      6.28. Haematite T/F?
(e)   **6.29.** Silica T/F?

Answers overleaf

6.20. T.

(v. inf.)

6.21. F.

6.22. T.

Both this and 6.20 result in inability to get rid of inspired micro-organisms which have been caught in the mucus film.

6.23. T.

Distal to the obstruction.

6.24. F.

Both this and 6.21 carry *some* increased risk of lung infection, but not "major" as with the other three.

6.25—29. All F.

Chiefly put in this form to show that there is no reason why a group of questions like this should not all be right or all wrong, though examiners usually avoid such extremes. But it is very hard to find a dust that does not cause lung disease if inhaled in sufficient quantities.

Beryllium produces a very peculiar sarcoidosis-like lesion.

6.30—35. Well recognized associations?

       6.30. Bronchiectasis and cerebral abscess T/F?
(e)   **6.31.** Carcinoma of bronchus and cerebral metastases T/F?
       6.32. Farmer's lung and fungal infection of brain T/F?
       6.33. Influenza and viral encephalitis T/F?
       6.34. Obstructed eustachian tube and cerebral abscess T/F?
       6.35. Primary tuberculous focus and meningitis T/F?

Answers overleaf

6.30. T.

6.31. T.

6.32. F.

Farmer's lung is a sensitization to fungal spores, not an infection.

6.33. F.

Direct effects of the influenza virus are very strictly limited to the respiratory tract.

6.34. T.

Via otitis media (perhaps a little remote!).

6.35. T.

By far the commonest fatal complication of primary tuberculosis in children is tuberculous meningitis.

7. ALIMENTARY SYSTEM

7.01—3. Usual behaviour of these tumours?

7.01. Mixed-salivary tumour of parotid gland (pleomorphic adenoma)

7.02. Squamous carcinoma of lip

7.03. Squamous carcinoma of pharynx

A. Benign, slow-growing
B. Fairly well differentiated, metastases usually late
C. Poorly differentiated, metastasizes rapidly (common in Chinese)
D. Rapidly growing but never metastasizes
E. Slow growing, often recurs locally, rarely metastasizes.

(e) 7.04. The common malignant tumour of the oesophagus is?

F. Adenocarcinoma
G. Myosarcoma
H. Papillary cystadenocarcinoma
J. Spheroidal-cell carcinoma
K. Squamous carcinoma.

7.05. There is a not very rare congenital anomaly in which the baby is born with a communication between oesophagus and trachea. If not discovered, this may be rapidly fatal, the cause of death being?

L. Bronchopneumonia
M. Dehydration
N. Oesophagitis
O. Pressure on superior vena cava
P. Starvation.

Answers overleaf

7.01. E.

7.02. B.

7.03. C.

Often a "lymphoepithelioma". Why? (See Deferred Notes.)

7.04. K.

As one would expect from its squamous lining.

7.05. L.

Due to passage of food into the trachea.

(e) 7.06. <u>*LEAST*</u> likely cause of haematemesis?

Q. Acute gastric ulcer
R. Atrophic gastritis
S. Carcinoma of stomach
T. Chronic gastric ulcer
U. Duodenal ulcer
V. Oesophageal varices.

7.07. The commonest and most important consequence of repeated small bleeds from a peptic ulcer over several years is?

V. Aplastic anaemia
W. Endarteritis obliterans
X. Iron deficiency anaemia
Y. Reduced blood volume
Z. Reduced plasma protein.

(e) 7.08. <u>*NOT*</u> one of the four major complications of peptic ulcer

A. Fibrous stricture
B. Haemorrhage
C. Imperfect digestion of food
D. Malignancy
E. Perforation.

7.09—11. Probable diagnosis in these ulcers of the stomach?

7.09. Punched out, on lesser curve, 20 mm. diam., penetrating muscle, fibrosis visible on outside

7.10. Punched out, on anterior wall, 10 mm. diam., shallow

7.11. Thick irregular rolled edges, near pylorus, 30 mm. diam.

F. Acute peptic ulcer
G. Carcinoma
H. Chronic peptic ulcer
J. Lymphosarcoma
K. Myoma.

Answers overleaf

7.06. R.

The question has been stretched to a one-from-six to include all five major causes of haematemesis: various haemorrhagic diseases might have been included also however. *Large* haemorrhages are not a common result of gastric cancers.

7.07. X.

The inevitable consequence of repeated haemorrhage, loss of iron being very difficult to replace. Y results from a single large haemorrhage.

7.08. C.

There is no failure of digestion, in the scientific sense of the word, in ulcer patients, however popular the word "indigestion" may be for pain due to the ulcer. You should in any case recognize the other four as true. But A and D both have limited distributions: that is to say, they do not complicate ulcers at all sites. Where are they found? (See Deferred Notes.)

7.09. H.

7.10. F.

7.11. G.

7.12. <u>*NOT*</u> likely to be found in the presence of severe atrophic gastritis

    L.   Duodenal ulcer
    M. Gastric carcinoma
    N. Gastric polyp
    O. Iron deficiency anaemia
    P. Pernicious anaemia.

7.13. *FOURTH* in this sequence?

    Q. Acute appendicitis
    R. Adhesion of ileum to caecum
    S. Intestinal obstruction
    T. Peritonitis in right iliac fossa
    U. Twisting of loop of ileum.

7.14. An elderly man who has had several attacks of coronary disease is admitted to hospital for incipient gangrene of one leg and found on admission to have symptoms of intestinal obstruction. What is the most probable cause of the latter?

    V. Cancer of colon
    W. Intussusception
    X. Mesenteric thrombosis
    Y. Strangulated hernia
    Z. Volvulus.

7.15. <u>*NOT*</u> characteristic of malabsorption syndrome (gluten enteropathy)

    A. Deficiency of disaccharidases in intestinal secretions
    B. Failure to absorb folic acid
    C. Flattening of villi in jejunum
    D. Low serum albumen
    E. Scanty dark-coloured faeces.

Answers overleaf

7.12. L.

Severe mucosal atrophy means almost certainly achlorhydria, which means any kind of peptic ulcer is very improbable.

7.13. U.

Sequence is Q, T, R, U, S — a typical history in a case of ileus due to adhesions.

7.14. X.

The rest are possible (though W is nearly excluded by age) but X relates to the rest of his history. How? (See Deferred Notes.)

7.15. E.

The bulky pale offensive faeces, full of unabsorbed fat, are usually an obvious clinical feature.

7.16. A patient who has been ill for four weeks with fever and diarrhoea dies suddenly. At post mortem general peritonitis is found, with perforation of the ileum. Peyer's patches are swollen and ulcerated and the spleen enlarged. You would suspect?

F. Bacillary dysentery
G. Gastroenteritis
H. Intestinal ischaemia
J. Typhoid
K. Tuberculous enteritis.

7.17. *NOT* characteristic of argentaffinoma (carcinoid) of the ileum?

L. Brown subnuclear granules stainable with silver
M. Excretion of catecholamines in the urine
N. Flushing attacks
O. Long survival even with metastases
P. Pulmonary stenosis.

7.18. *FOURTH* in this sequence?

Q. Cystitis
R. Diverticula of colon
S. Diverticulitis
T. Pericolic abscess
U. Vesico-colic fistula.

7.19. *NOT* characteristic of Crohn's disease?

V. Cobblestone appearance of mucosa
W. Commonest site is the jejunum
X. Fistulas frequent
Y. May involve colon
Z. Oedematous thickening of one or more segments of bowel.

Answers overleaf

7.16. J.

The Peyer's patch distribution strongly indicates it, and the history is typical. Or paratyphoid, of course.

7.17. M.

Argentaffinoma cases excrete 5-hydroxy-indole acetic acid: catecholamines indicate phaeochromocytoma.

7.18. U.

Sequence is R, S, T, U, Q. Formation of a fistula from colon to bladder in this way is not rare.

7.19. W.

Ileum, not jejunum (hence 'regional ileitis'), though lesions may be found almost anywhere in the gut.

(e) 7.20. The common malignant tumour of the large intestine is:

- A. Adenocarcinoma
- B. Adenomatous polyp
- C. Lymphosarcoma
- D. Melanoma
- E. Squamous carcinoma.

7.21. If at operation on a man of 55 the whole pyloric half of the stomach is found to have its wall 2—3 cm. thick and very firm, the most probable diagnosis is:

- F. Congenital pyloric stenosis
- G. Gumma
- H. Healed gastric ulcer
- J. Phlegmonous gastritis
- K. Scirrhous carcinoma.

7.22. If you find in the colon irregular ulcers with little inflammation and deeply undermined edges, and the patient has recently come from the tropics, which protozoon might you suspect?

- L. *Entamoeba histolytica*
- M. *Leishmania donovani*
- N. *Plasmodium vivax*
- O. *Toxoplasma gondii*
- P. *Trypanosoma gambiense.*

7.23—25. Most probable cause of obstructions at these sites?

7.23. First part of duodenum	Q. Carcinoma
7.24. Ileum	R. Crohn's disease
7.25. Sigmoid colon	S. Pressure from enlarged lymph nodes
	T. Peptic ulcer
	Y. Syphilis.

Answers overleaf

7.20. A.

B is probably commoner, but not malignant.

7.21. K.

The so-called "leather-bottle" appearance, which nowadays practically always means scirrhous carcinoma.

7.22. L.

This might be amoebic dysentery. What do the other protozoa cause? (See Deferred Notes.)

7.23. T.

Pyloric stenosis due to duodenal ulcer: despite its name the stricture is actually in the duodenum, though its effect is the same as that of a true pyloric stenosis.

7.24. R.

7.25. Q.

7.26. Unusually persistent recurrence of peptic ulcers suggests the possibility of?

V. Adrenal cortical adenoma
W. Basophile adenoma of the pituitary
X. Hepatoma
Y. Medullary carcinoma of the thyroid
Z. Pancreatic islet-cell tumour.

7.27. The one *certain* known factor in the aetiology of peptic ulcer is the constant presence of:

A. Acid gastric juice
B. Anxiety
C. Blood group A
D. Hypermotility
E. Vagal over-activity.

(e) 7.28. Complicates gastric ulcer but never duodenal?

F. Haematemesis
G. Malignancy
H. Melaena
J. Perforation
K. Stenosis.

7.29. In congenital megacolon of the Hirschsprung's type the essential lesion is:

L. Exaggerated sacculation
M. Loss of ganglion cells over a short segment
N. Partially imperforate anus
O. Stenosis of rectum
P. Weakness of taeniae coli and circular muscle.

Answers overleaf

7.26. Z.

The gastrin-secreting type (Zollinger-Ellison syndrome), not the insulin-secreting type.

7.27. A.

Peptic ulcer only occurs in areas bathed by acid. Other factors are often present, but nothing like as constantly.

7.28. G.

Malignancy of any kind is rare in the duodenum.

7.29. M.

Failure of peristalsis in the affected segment leads to dilatation of the colon above the segment.

(e) 7.30. Usual consequence of obstruction of the common bile duct?

Q. Jaundice with dark urine and dark stools
R. Jaundice with dark urine and pale stools
S. Jaundice with pale urine and dark stools
T. Jaundice with pale urine and pale stools
U. No jaundice.

7.31. If a gall-bladder contains a single large pale stone, seen on section to consist of radiating pale yellow or white translucent crystals, it almost certainly consists of?

V. Calcium carbonate
W. Cholesterol
X. Cystine
Y. Pigment
Z. Uric acid.

(e) 7.32. *NOT* a possible effect on the gall-bladder of long-continued obstruction of its neck by a stone?

A. Acute cholecystitis
B. Cancer
C. Distension with bile
D. Fibrous constriction
E. Mucocele.

7.33. *FOURTH* in this sequence?

F. Cholecystitis
G. Liver failure
H. Multiple pigmented stones in gall-bladder
J. Stone in common bile duct
K. Suppurative cholangitis.

Answers overleaf

7.30. R.

This is a kind of *pons asinorum* in pathology. If you chose any other answer, go away and read it up until you know not only the right answer, but *why* it is the right answer.

7.31. W.

The commonest solitary stone, even without the evidence of the appearance.

7.32. C.

How can bile enter a gall-bladder with an obstructed neck, let alone distend it?

7.33. K.

The sequence is F, H, J, K, G.

7.34. *FOURTH* in this sequence?

    L. Acute cholecystitis
    M. Cellulitis around portal fissure
    N. Haematemesis
    O. Oesophageal varices
    P. Thrombosis of portal vein.

(e) 7.35. In acute pancreatitis the diagnosis may be established by the presence in the blood of an excess of which enzyme?

    Q. Acid phosphatase
    R. Alkaline phosphatase
    S. Amylase
    T. Creatine kinase
    U. Transaminases.

7.36. *NOT* a common complication of carcinoma of the pancreas?

    V. Blocked-duct atrophy of pancreas
    W. Dilatation of pancreatic ducts to form a single large cyst
    X. Increased tendency to venous thrombosis
    Y. Metastases in liver
    Z. Obstructive jaundice.

7.37. Describes fibrocystic disease of the pancreas?

    A. Congenital disorder of secretion of multiple glands
    B. Cystic malformation of pancreas
    C. Late result of acute pancreatitis
    D. Secretory defect limited to pancreas
    E. Unexplained pancreatic disease seen chiefly in middle-aged men.

Answers overleaf

7.34. O.

The sequence is L, M, P, O, N. Not common, but logical enough: and a reminder that portal vein thrombosis can imitate the vascular effects of cirrhosis.

7.35. S.

Since this is secreted by the pancreas. What diseases do you associate with the other enzymes? (See Deferred Notes.)

7.36. W.

All the others are very common. Formation of single cysts is only common with duct blockage in *small* glands — Bartholin's is the largest in which it happens.

7.37. A.

There are defects of secretion of salivary, bronchial and intestinal glands as well as pancreas (hence "mucoviscidosis") and an excess of sodium in the sweat.

(e) 7.38. The commonest acute infection of the liver is?

F. Brucellosis
G. Infective hepatitis
H. Leptospirosis
J. Serum hepatitis
K. Suppurative cholangitis.

(e) 7.39. Detection of the Australia antigen is of importance chiefly in the prevention of:

L. Cholangiolytic hepatitis
M. Infective hepatitis
N. Q fever
O. Serum hepatitis
P. Toxoplasmosis.

7.40. Viral hepatitis is particularly dangerous in?

Q. Females in late teens
R. Males in late teens
S. Post-menopausal women
T. School children
U. Sedentary middle-aged men.

(e) 7.41. _NOT_ a consequence of advanced cirrhosis of the liver?

V. Ascites
W. Gall stones
X. Hepatoma
Y. Liver failure
Z. Rupture of oesophageal varices producing haematemesis.

Answers overleaf

7.38. G.

In its milder forms a very common infection.

7.39. O.

Detection allows for instance the elimination of many potential carriers from blood donors.

7.40. S.

They are particularly liable to develop chronic active hepatitis.

7.41. W.

Gall stones can occasionally *cause* cirrhosis (of biliary type) but are not a consequence of it. The other four are the major complications of cirrhosis.

(e) 7.42. The commonest malignant tumour to be found in the liver at post mortem is?

    A. Angiosarcoma
    B. Cholangiocarcinoma
    C. Hepatoblastoma
    D. Hepatoma
    E. Metastatic carcinoma.

7.43—45. In which category of cirrhosis would you place these?

    7.43. The largest number of cases of cirrhosis in the U.K.

    7.44. A liver of about normal size, with nodules averaging about 1 mm. diameter, yellow and greasy to touch

    7.45. A large liver, finely nodular, deep green in colour.

    F. Alcoholic
    G. Biliary
    H. Post-hepatitic
    J. Nutritional
    K. Unknown cause.

7.46. The combination at post mortem of a massively enlarged black liver and a glass eye suggests?

    L. Argyria
    M. Chronic malaria
    N. Hepato-lenticular degeneration
    O. Melanoma of eye
    P. Melanosis coli.

7.47. *NOT* proved experimentally to cause cancer of the liver?

    Q. Aflatoxin (from groundnuts)
    R. Butter yellow
    S. Carbon tetrachloride
    T. Colloidal carbon
    U. Senecio alkaloids.

Answers overleaf

7.42. E.

Much commoner than any primary. If one had said "of the" instead of "in the" liver, D would have been the answer.

7.43. K.

Surprising, but true: cases with no known cause amount to at least 50% of all cases of cirrhosis.

7.44. F.

A fatty liver with cirrhosis is usually alcoholic.

7.45. G.

Also typical. Other kinds of cirrhosis are rarely deeply bile stained. (The green staining is only well developed in fixed specimens: in life bile-stained organs are orange in colour).

7.46. O.

Rare, but a classical combination, often missed clinically. The liver is of course full of secondaries. The eye may have been removed many years earlier. (The lens of hepato-lenticular degeneration is of course the lentiform nucleus).

7.47. T.

This will be taken up by the Kupffer cells, but causes no permanent damage.

7.48 —52. Relatively common consequences of severe multi-lobular cirrhosis of the liver?

   7.48. Atrophy of testes T/F?

   7.49. Low serum albumen T/F?

   7.50. Prolonged deep jaundice T/F?

   7.51. Raised serum globulin T/F?

   7.52. Subacute combined degeneration of the spinal cord T/F?

Answers overleaf

7.48. T.

Due to failure of inactivation of oestrogen, a normal liver function.

7.49. T.

Due to failure of manufacture.

7.50. F.

Unusual except of course in biliary cirrhosis.

7.51. T.

7.52. F.

8. GENITO-URINARY SYSTEMS

Urinary

(e) 8.01. A stone firmly lodged in the right ureter will cause uraemia if?

    A. Left kidney is absent
    B. Patient is already hypertensive
    C. Right kidney shows severe pyonephrosis
    D. Severe cystitis is present
    E. Stone is exceptionally large.

8.02—4. Most probable cause of oedema occurring in different forms of glomerulonephritis?

8.02. Acute diffuse	F. Heart failure due to hypertension
8.03. Subacute progressive	G. Increased capillary permeability
	H. Inferior vena cava thrombosis
8.04. Chronic	J. Low serum albumin due to heavy loss in urine
	K. Thiamine deficiency.

(e) 8.05. The single most useful test to determine the presence of kidney disease is?

    L. Addis count (of cells in urine)
    M. Blood urea
    N. Creatinine clearance
    O. Excretory pyelogram
    P. Urine albumen.

Answers overleaf

8.01. A.

In such circumstances the crucial factor is the function of the *other* kidney.

8.02. G.

8.03. J.

This applies to any kidney disease producing heavy albuminuria — such as? (See Deferred Notes.)

8.04. F.

Oedema is not in fact an important complication — the polyuria tends to produce dehydration if anything.

8.05. P.

This is a poor question but good propaganda. Speaking as a pathologist, one far too often sees patients at post mortem with pages of biochemistry but no record of the urine albumen.

8.06. In a case of chronic glomerulonephritis in the early stages of renal failure (i.e. with a moderately raised blood urea and mild hypertension) you would expect to find the urine?

  Q. Increased in volume, with fixed low Sp.G. and a trace of albumen.
  R. Much increased in volume, with high Sp.G. and no albumen
  S. Normal except for heavy albuminuria
  T. Normal except for low volume
  U. Normal except for albumen and very numerous pus cells.

(e) 8.07—11. Characteristic of acute diffuse glomerulonephritis?

  8.07. Crescents in glomeruli T/F?
  8.08. Damage to glomeruli probably due to antigen-antibody complexes T/F?
  8.09. Decreased urine output T/F?
  8.10. Related infection is usually type 12 streptococcus T/F?
  8.11. Related infection occurs nearly simultaneously with onset T/F?

Answers overleaf

8.06. Q.

This type of urine output is very characteristic of renal failure due to loss of the majority of nephrons, however caused. What could be the cause of the other types of urine? (See Deferred Notes.)

8.07. F.

Glomeruli are swollen, with polymorphs. Crescents occur in subacute progressive form.

8.08. T.

8.09. T.

8.10. T.

8.11. F.

Onset *follows* the infection, by an average of 10 days — as one would expect with an immuno-reaction.

8.12—17. Diseases in which renal failure accounts for a substantial proportion of the fatal cases?

(e) 8.12. Amyloidosis T/F?
(e) 8.13. Diabetes insipidus T/F?
    8.14. Diabetes mellitus T/F?
    8.15. Gout T/F?
    8.16. Mismatched transfusion T/F?
    8.17. Smallpox T/F

8.18—22. Characteristic of clear-cell carcinoma of kidney ("hypernephroma")?

    8.18. Cannon ball metastasis in lung T/F?
    8.19. Common in aniline dye workers T/F?
    8.20. Frequently arises from mesonephric tissues outside kidney T/F?
    8.21. High glycogen content T/F?
    8.22. Solitary bone metastases. T/F?

Answers overleaf

8.12. T.

Amyloid kidney is the principal danger of amyloidosis.

8.13. F.

8.14. T.

Kimmelstiel-Wilson kidney, medullary necrosis and increased liability to urinary infections all contribute.

8.15. T.

8.16. T.

Pigment nephropathy produces acute renal failure.

8.17. F.

8.18. T.

8.19. F.

No known aetiology: but dye workers may have tumours of renal *pelvis* as well as bladder.

8.20. F.

8.21. T.

8.22. T.

8.18 and 8.22 perhaps associated with tendency to macroscopic renal vein involvement.

8.23—26. Concerning some miscellaneous renal diseases.

8.23. Disseminated lupus erythematosus: the characteristic kidney lesion is loss of pedicels on E.M. T/F?

8.24. Malignant hypertension: shows fibrinoid necrosis (fibrinous vasculosis) in the efferent arterioles T/F?

8.25. Symmetrical cortical necrosis: chiefly seen in post-partum haemorrhage T/F?

8.26. Transplanted kidney patients: liable to opportunistic infections T/F?

Male genital

8.26. When tuberculosis affects the male genital tract, it usually first appears in?

V. Epididymis
W. Prostate
X. Seminal vesicles
Y. Testis
Z. Urethra.

8.27. The common chromosomal defect that causes testicular atrophy and male sterility is?

A. Mosaicism
B. Translocation
C. XO (Turner's syndrome)
D. XXY (Klinefelter's syndrome)
E. XYY.

8.28 *NOT* true of seminoma of the testis?

F. Arises in epididymis as often as testis proper
G. Commonest in young adult males
H. Has a better prognosis than teratoma of the testis
J. Peculiarly radiosensitive
K. Relatively commoner in undescended than descended testis.

Answers overleaf

8.23. F.

Wireloops: pedicel lesions may be seen, but are not characteristic, being present in any variety of the nephrotic syndrome.

8.24. F.

Afferent arterioles: lesions of efferents seen only in diabetes mellitus.

8.25. T.

The massive shut-down of much of the cortical blood flow in reaction to shock (which causes CN) is for some unknown reason especially likely to occur in pregnancy.

8.26. T.

A consequence of immunosuppressive treatment.

8.26. V.

It may spread to the others secondarily. Syphilis, in contrast, affects the external genitalia in the primary form and the testis in gummas.

8.27. D.

XO produces *female* infertility.

8.28. F.

Almost entirely confined to the testis.

8.29—32. Complications of cases of enlarged prostate (benign prostatomegaly, benign nodular hyperplasia):

8.29. Carcinoma of the periurethral part of the prostate T/F?
8.30. Cystitis T/F?
8.31. Transitional-cell carcinoma of the renal pelvis T/F?
8.32. Uraemia T/F?

Female genital

8.33. A corpus luteum is seen in one of the ovaries in:

L. First half of normal menstrual cycle only
M. Second half of normal menstrual cycle only
N. Pregnancy
O. Both L and M
P. Both M and N

8.34. A massive haemorrhage into the pelvic peritoneum is most likely to be due to?

Q. Ectopic pregnancy
R. Endometriosis
S. Menorrhagia
T. Missed abortion
U. Salpingitis.

8.35. Tubercles in endometrial curettings indicate?

V. Miliary tuberculosis
W. Non-specific inflammation
X. Sarcoidosis
Y. Tuberculosis of the fallopian tube
Z. Tuberculosis of the lung.

Answers overleaf

8.29. F.

Malignancy does occur, but it involves the compressed peripheral part of the gland, especially the posterior surface.

8.30. T.

8.31. F.

8.32. T.

A result of renal damage due to back-pressure and infection.

8.33. P.

Strictly speaking the CL of the previous cycle is still present during much of the next cycle, but in process of atrophy: its active phase is confined to the 7—10 days after ovulation.

8.34. Q.

Associated with extrusion of the pregnancy from the fallopian tube or rupture of the tube.

8.35. Y.

Other forms of tuberculosis, such as V or Z, may well be present, but the immediate pointer is to the tube, from which tubercle bacilli are being discharged into the uterus. This used to be very common, and an important cause of sterility.

8.36. Complication of post-partum haemorrhage that can give rise to amenorrhoea and sterility?

    A.   Amniotic fluid embolism
    B.   Bronchopneumonia
    C.   Cortical necrosis of kidney
    D.   Iliac vein thrombosis
    E.   Pituitary necrosis (Sheehan's disease).

(e) 8.37. The commonest benign tumour of the female genital tract is the?

    F.   Brenner tumour of ovary
    G.   Endocervical polyp
    H.   Mucinous cystadenoma of ovary
    J.   Myoma of uterus
    K.   Serous cystadenoma of ovary.

(e) 8.38. The principal object of the screening of large numbers of women by cervical cytology tests is to reduce the the incidence of cancer of the cervix by catching cases at the stage of?

    L.   Carcinoma-in-situ
    M.   Dysplasia
    N.   Epidermidization
    O.   Erosion
    P.   Stage I cancer.

(e) 8.39. Ninety per cent of carcinomas of the cervix are?

    Q.   Adenocarcinoma
    R.   Clear-cell carcinoma
    S.   Papillary cystadenocarcinoma
    T.   Spheroid-cell carcinoma
    U.   Squamous carcinoma.

Answers overleaf

8.36. E.

Haemorrhage $\longrightarrow$ Shock $\longrightarrow$ (especially in pregnancy) necrosis of pituitary (or kidney or spleen) $\longrightarrow$ failure of FSH etc. $\longrightarrow$ no ovulation.

8.37. J.

One of the commonest of all tumours. G is also common, but is not a tumour.

8.38. L.

P is too late, M, N, and O are common conditions with little association with cancer.

8.39. U.

They arise mostly from the unstable edge of the squamous epithelium where it meets the columnar epithelium.
Ten per cent arise from the latter, and are adenocarcinomas.

8.40—42. Characteristics of these ovarian tumours?

8.40. Dysgerminoma	V. Analogue of seminoma of testis
8.41. Granulosa cell tumour	
8.42. Mucinous cystadeno-carcinoma.	W. Full of butter-like material
	X. Never metastasizes
	Y. Secretes oestrogens
	Z. Spread often limited to peritoneum for long time.

8.43—46. A woman dies in a car accident the day after an uneventful therapeutic abortion in which the material passed included a 2½ month normal foetus. Findings at post mortem would be expected to include?

8.43. Chorionic villi in the implantation site containing both syncytiotrophoblast and cytotrophoblast T/F?
8.44. Ditto, containing vessels with nucleated red cells T/F?
8.45. Decidual reaction of the remaining endometrium T/F?
8.46. No corpus luteum in either ovary T/F?

Breast

8.47. A tumour forming a solitary spherical lump in the otherwise normal breast of a woman of 28 is probably?

A. Adenoma
B. Carcinoma
C. Fibroadenoma
D. Fibrocystic disease
E. Fibroma.

Answers overleaf

8.40. V.

Histologically similar, and both arise often from abnormal gonads.

8.41. Y.

8.42. Z.

W would of course fit a dermoid cyst: X would fit a Brenner tumour or a parovarian cyst if the "never" were relaxed a little.

8.43. T.

As in early pregnancy. Some villi nearly always remain in the uterus for a short time after abortion — sometimes longer.

8.44. T.

As in any pregnancy except near term.

8.45. T.

As in any pregnancy.

8.46. F.

A CL of pregnancy would be present. For this and the preceding findings, relatively little change occurs in the tissues remaining during the twenty four hours after an abortion.

8.47. C.

A and E are rare, B uncommon at this age (but *cannot* be eliminated without biopsy), D is not a tumour.

8.48. The real argument for doing rapid frozen (cryostat) sections on all breast lumps before completing the operation?

    F.   Cryostat section diagnosis is 100% certain in all cases

    G.   It enables one to distinguish between scirrhous and encephaloid cancers

    H.   It is medicolegally mandatory

    J.   No surgeon can ever confidently diagnose a cancer of the breast without histology

    K.   The increased certainty of diagnosis in most cases greatly outweighs the inconvenience of the procedure.

8.49. The man who discovered the relationship between a disease of the nipple and cancer of the breast described another condition that also bears his name?

    L.   A bone disease of the elderly

    M.   A form of cirrhosis

    N.   A primary tumour of lymph nodes

    O.   Chronic nephritis

    P.   Multiple tumours of nerves.

8.50–54. Carcinoma of the breast is:

(e)   8.50. Commoner in this country than any of the cancers of the femal genital tract T/F?

(e)   8.51. Spread chiefly by the lymphatics T/F?

        8.52. Sometimes hormone-dependent T/F?

        8.53. The usual consequence when a fibroadenoma goes malignant T/F?

        8.54. Very rare in the male breast T/F?

Answers overleaf

8.48. K.

G is also true, but not much practical help: none of the others is true, though on medicolegal grounds it is certainly advisable where possible.

8.49. L.

Paget, a London surgeon, 1814—1899. What are the other eponyms? (See Deferred Notes.)

8.50. T.

(Cervix is commoner in countries of very high birthrate.)

8.51. T.

8.52. T.

8.53. F.

When (rarely) this happens, the result is usually a sarcoma.

8.54. F.

Uncommon (1% of breast ca) but not rare.

9. MISCELLANEOUS (A)

Endocrines

(e) **9.01. Destruction of the pituitary stalk and the neighbouring part of the hypothalamus usually produces which alteration in the urine?**

    A. Constant mild albuminuria
    B. Glycosuria (sugar)
    C. Intermittent heavy albuminuria
    D. Oliguria (too little)
    E. Polyuria (too much).

9.02—4. Probable diagnosis with given histology of enlarged thyroid gland?

    9.02. Colloid abundant, solid-looking, epithelial cells flattened

    9.03. Reduced colloid, often watery, epithelial cells tall columnar

    9.04. Small acini often with no colloid, epithelial cells large and pink-staining, masses of lymphocytes and plasma cells.

    F. Cretinism
    G. Goitre of iodine deficiency type
    H. Hashimoto's disease
    J. Hyperthyroidism
    K. Lymphosarcoma.

Answers overleaf

9.01. E.

This is diabetes insipidus, produced by lack of ADH due to destruction of the hypothalamic nuclei that produce it.

9.02. G.

This is colloid goitre, which *can* be due to iodine deficiency.

9.03. J.

Signs of increased secretion.

9.04. H.

The acini show evidence of damage by autoimmune reaction, and the dense cellular infiltrate round them is part of this reaction.

9.05. In severe and long-standing chronic uraemia you would expect the parathyroids to be?

   L.   All enlarged
   M. All reduced in size
   N.   Normal
   O.   Normal in size, but calcified
   P.   One replaced by adenoma, rest normal in size.

(e) 9.06. *NOT* a characteristic consequence of destruction of both adrenals?

   Q. Addison's disease
   R. High blood sodium
   S.   Low blood pressure
   T.   Pigmentation of skin
   U. Weakness of muscles.

9.07—9. In three cases of hypertension due to adrenal lesions, urinary findings were as indicated. Which adrenal lesion do they suggest?

9.07. Glycosuria	V. Adaptation syndrome
9.08. High catecholamines	W. Adrenogenital
9.09. Raised urinary output of	syndrome
potassium, lowered out-	X. Conn's syndrome
put of sodium.	Y. Cushing's syndrome
	Z. Phaeochromocytoma.

9.10—12. Each of the following can be produced by a disease of some endocrine gland. Identify for each a consequence of another disease of the same gland.

9.10. Exophthalmos	A. Kidney stones
9.11. Ulcers of stomach	B. Mental defect
9.12. Virilization	(congenital)
	C. Pulmonary stenosis
	D. Sudden collapse in
	meningococcal
	septicaemia
	E. Sudden giddiness and
	loss of consciousness.

Answers overleaf

9.05. L.

This is secondary hyperparathyroidism, a reaction to phosphate retention by the failing kidney. P is of course the adenoma of primary hyperparathyroidism.

9.06. R.

The *low* blood sodium of Addison's disease is one of the most important features of the disease.

9.07. Y.

Result of excessive production of glucocorticoid steroids.

9.08. Z.

This tumour of adrenal medulla secretes chiefly noradrenaline, which produces hypertension and is excreted as catecholamines.

9.09. X.

Result of excessive production of aldosterone. The urine outputs would reflect sodium retention and potassium loss: in practice the crude levels of output would probably not mean much without relation to blood levels.

9.10. B.

Thyroid, with hyperthyroidism and congenital atrophy (cretinism).

9.11. E.

Islets of Langhans, with gastrin-producing and insulin-producing tumours respectively.

9.12. D.

Adrenal, with adreno-genital syndrome and Waterhouse-Friderichsen syndrome of adrenal necrosis.

9.13—17. Characteristic of carcinoma of the thyroid:

        9.13. Especially rare in iodine-deficiency areas T/F?

(e)   **9.14.** May obstruct the trachea T/F?

        9.15. Often metastasizes to bone T/F?

        9.16. Often produces hyperthyroidism T/F?

        9.17. Papillary form an important complication of radiation of the neck in childhood T/F?

9.18—21. Destruction of the anterior pituitary in an adult produces:

(e)   **9.18.** Adrenal atrophy T/F?

(e)   **9.19.** Cystic disease of breast T/F?

(e)   **9.20.** Goitre T/F?

        9.21. Maldescent of testis T/F?

Answers overleaf

9.13. F.

Cancer is commoner with most forms of goitre than with normal glands.

9.14. T.

As might be expected from the anatomy.

9.15. T.

9.16. F.

Surprisingly rarely, in fact.

9.17. T.

Thyroid in childhood is peculiarly susceptible to irradiation, and papillary tumour in the teens is the usual result.

9.18. T.

(ACTH lack.)

9.19. F.

Simple atrophy.

9.20. F.

(TSH lack.)

9.21. F.

Atrophy occurs, but will not affect position of a testis already descended.

(Hormones concerned in 19 and 21 still controversial.)

9.22. Part of a lymph node associated with thymic lymphocytes?

F. Deep cortex
G. Germ centres
H. Peripheral sinus
J. Radial sinus
K. Superficial cortex.

9.23. Calcified lymph nodes in the mesentery ("tabes mesenterica") are nearly always a consequence of?

L. Lymphatic spread of tuberculosis from lungs
M. Pancreatitis with fat necrosis
N. Primary tuberculosis of ileum in childhood
O. Secondary carcinoma
P. Toxoplasmosis.

9.24. In a patient clinically thought to have Hodgkin's disease an excised lymph node proves to be packed with tubercles, consisting of epithelioid cells and giant cells with no caseation. No AFB are found, and the tuberculin test is negative. Probable diagnosis?

Q. Hodgkin's disease
R. Reticulosarcoma
S. Sarcoidosis
T. Syphilis
U. Toxoplasmosis.

9.25. Actually a very much enlarged lymph node?

V. Bubo of bubonic plague
W. Chancre of syphilis
X. Delhi boil of leishmaniasis
Y. Leproma of leprosy
Z. Malignant pustule of anthrax.

Answers overleaf

9.22. F.

This is the area that is deficient in mice whose thymus is removed soon after birth: also called "paracortical".

9.23. N.

A kind of 'primary complex' (primary focus in ileum, secondary focus in lymph nodes) that is usually derived from infected milk.

M produces calcification in the fat of the mesentery and P of the brain (in the congenital form).

9.24. S.

This tuberculosis-like histology without caseation is very characteristic of sarcoidosis, though it is not safe to eliminate tuberculosis on histology alone and there are other rarer pitfalls.

9.25. V.

Usually in the groin, from infected bites of rat fleas on the legs. All the others are usually lesions of the skin.

9.26—29. Characteristic of Hodgkin's disease:

> **9.26.** Affects especially children and the elderly T/F?
> **9.27.** Occurs in several forms of different degrees of malignancy T/F?
> **9.28.** Often terminates as leukaemia T/F?
> **9.29.** Special form of giant cells practically always present T/F?

9.30. Taking the world as a whole, the commonest cause of a really big spleen (1,000 g. or more) is?

> A. Amyloid
> B. Chronic myeloid leukaemia
> C. Cirrhosis of liver
> D. Gaucher's disease
> E. Malaria.

9.31. _NOT_ regularly associated with an enlarged spleen?

> F. Congestive heart failure
> G. Haemolytic anaemia
> H. Malabsorption
> J. Obstruction of portal vein
> K. Right heart failure.

Answers overleaf

9.26. F.

Maximum incidence in middle life.

9.27. T.

The names change every few years: students are advised to content themselves with the names currently favoured by their local pathology department.

9.28. F.

Only lymphosarcoma has any substantial tendency to leukaemia.

9.29. T.

The Reed-Sternberg mirror-image giant cells should always be demonstrated before making the diagnosis, but they may be scanty.

9.30. E.

Malaria is still very common over vast areas of the world. All the other conditions produce big spleens, but none are so common. In cirrhosis, the commonest, a 1,000 g. spleen is unusual. If one confined the question to the U.K. the answer would probably be B.

9.31. H.

The spleen is often very small in malabsorption. (A rather recondite answer, but it is hard to find plausible conditions in which the spleen is *not* enlarged: one would expect most people to arrive at it by exclusion — all the rest are well-known causes of enlargement.)

9.32. If one divides the haematocrit reading on a sample of blood by the red cell count, and makes the appropriate adjustment in decimal point and units, one has calculated?

   L. Mean corpuscular haemoglobin
   M. Mean corpuscular haemoglobin concentration
   N. Mean red cell volume
   O. Red cell diameter
   P. Red cell thickness.

(e) 9.33. The commonest microcytic hypochromic anaemia?

   Q. Acholuric jaundice
   R. Aplastic anaemia
   S. Iron deficiency
   T. Pernicious anaemia
   U. Thalassaemia.

9.34. *FOURTH* element in this sequence of causation of pernicious anaemia?

   V. Atrophic gastritis
   W. Autoimmune reaction to gastric parietal cells
   X. Deficiency of intrinsic factor secretion
   Y. Failure to absorb cyanocobalamine
   Z. Prevention of maturation of red cell precursors in marrow.

9.35. Seven days after a single massive bleed from an oesophageal varix in a patient whose blood had previously been normal, what new feature would you expect to see in the red cells?

   A. Increased size
   B. Decreased size
   C. Increased haemoglobin content per cell
   D. Decreased haemoglobin content per cell
   E. Reticulocyte increase.

Answers overleaf

9.32. N.

If one begins with one mm^3 of blood, the haematocrit reading (expressed as a fraction rather than a percentage) gives the total volume of the red cells in that blood. Dividing that by the number of red cells in the same cubic millimetre obviously gives the volume per red cell. E.g. for normal values: Haematocrit 0.45 ÷ red count 5,000,000 per mm^3 = 0.00000009 mm^3 = 90 μm^3.

9.33. S.

Iron lack leads to lack of haemoglobin, so there is too low a concentration of haemoglobin (hypochromic) and the cells are reduced in both volume and diameter (microcytic).

9.34. Y.

The order is W, V, X, Y, Z.

9.35. E.

This is the mark of increased multiplication in the marrow to replace the lost red cells, the reticulocytes being the new young cells. At this stage the majority of the cells present are the survivors of the bleed, which remain normal in size and colour.

(What common form of treatment might *suppress* the reticulocyte reaction — see Deferred Notes.)

9.36. A boy whose tooth socket will not stop bleeding is known to have unaffected parents but a brother and a maternal uncle with similar trouble. Where is the defect likely to be?

F. Albumen
G. Capillaries
H. Fibrinogen
J. Globulin
K. Platelets

9.37. A blood donor of group A can give blood only to patients who are?

L. A or AB
M. A or AB or B
N. A or B or O
O. AB or O
P. B or O.

9.38—42. Factors whose deficiency causes clinically important anaemia in man:

　　9.38. Folic acid T/F?
(e)　**9.39.** Iron T/F?
(e)　**9.40.** Kallikrein T/F?
　　9.41. Vit. B_1 T/F?
(e)　**9.42.** Vit. B_{12} T/F?

9.43—45. If an Rh — ve woman has an affected baby in her first pregnancy it follows almost certainly that:

　　9.43. She must have had a previous transfusion of Rh +ve blood T/F?
　　9.44. Her husband must be Rh +ve T/F?
　　9.45. All subsequent pregnancies will be affected T/F?

Answers overleaf

9.36. J.

This is a typical history of haemophilia, in which the material missing is antihaemophilic globulin, an essential clotting factor. What can you say with certainty about the boy's mother? (See Deferred Notes.)

9.37. L.

Think of it *either* as donation to self and to universal recipient, *or* to anyone who also carries the allele A.

9.38. T, 9.39. T, 9.40. F, 9.41. F, 9.42. T.

None of these three "trues" is quite simply a deficiency in the sense in which scurvy is due to dietetic deficiency of Vit. C. With iron and folic acid there are usually excessive demands, and in both there may be and with B_{12} there always is defective absorption.

9.43. T.

Sensitization in a first pregnancy is otherwise very rare.

9.44. T.

Otherwise the child could not be Rhesus positive.

9.45. F.

If the father is heterozygous, there is an even chance that any subsequent child will be negative and hence unaffected. Prophylactic treatment might have the same effect, even if the child was positive.

9.46—48. Some characteristics of haemolytic anaemia:

(e) 9.46. Red marrow increased in bulk and cellularity T/F?
(e) 9.47. Red cell survival as measured by tagging with radio-chromium is increased T/F?
9.48. Urine generally normal T/F?

9.49—52. Concerning leukaemia:

(e) 9.49. The acute forms occur chiefly in children T/F?
9.50. Chronic myeloid leukaemia cells nearly always show a specific chromosome abnormality T/F?
9.51. Chronic lymphatic leukaemia occurs chiefly in young adults T/F?
9.52. Leukaemia caused by a virus occurs in domestic cats T/F?

Answers overleaf

9.46. T.

As required by continued need for more red cells.

9.47. F.

Cells are being destroyed too soon.

9.48. F.

Normal to look at (in contrast to obstructive jaundice) but excess of stercobilinogen in faeces leads to reabsorption and excretion as excess urobilinogen in urine.

9.49. T.

9.50. T.

The Philadelphia chromosome — deletion of half the long arm of chromosome 22 (or possible 21 — nomenclature is not quite certain: but not the same as the mongol chromosome as was once thought. It seems also now that it is not a deletion at all, but some kind of translocation).

9.51. F.

A disease chiefly of the elderly.

9.52. T.

A fairly recent discovery, but most animal leukaemias seem to be viral in origin, man being an apparent exception still, at least at the time of writing.

10. MISCELLANEOUS (B)

Locomotor

10.01. In "battered babies" subperiosteal haemorrhages in multiple bones, due to trauma, are often a prominent feature. With which bone disease might these lesions be confused?

   A. Hyperparathyroidism
   B. Pyogenic osteomyelitis
   C. Rickets
   D. Scurvy
   E. Vit. D poisoning.

10.02. The callus of an average well-splinted fracture at a stage when its shadow is conspicuous on an X-ray consists chiefly of?

   F. Calcified cartilage
   G. Calcified fibrin
   H. Compact lamellar bone
   J. Granulation tissue
   K. Irregularly arranged woven bone.

10.03. <u>NOT</u> a factor that promotes fracture healing?

   L. Absence of infection
   M. Adequate ascorbic acid
   N. Good blood supply
   O. Immobilization
   P. Treatment with cortisone.

Answers overleaf

10.01. D.

Haemorrhage under the periosteum is common in severe Vit. C deficiency. Easy bruising, and the fact that battered babies are often malnourished, increase the possibility of difficulty in diagnosis.

10.02. K.

Callus is real bone, though of the relatively ill-organized woven type. Some cases may however have a considerable admixture of cartilage, which is the major component of callus in some species such as mice.

10.03. P.

The adrenocortical steroids depress healing, though in practice it appears that only very high doses have much effect on fracture healing in man.

10.04. When the density of the shadow of a patch of bone is decreasing, the process occurring within bone nearly always involves?

    Q. Autolysis of bone
    R. Chemical removal of calcium salts from intact bone matrix
    S. Multiplication of osteoblasts
    T. Polymorph infiltration
    U. Resorption by osteoclasts.

10.05. _NOT_ characteristic of cases of extensive involvement of bone by secondary carcinoma?

    V. Both bone destruction and new bone formation possible
    W. Nucleated red cells often appear in peripheral blood
    X. Pathological fractures occur
    Y. Rise in blood alkaline phosphatase usual
    Z. Yellow marrow areas affected more than red marrow.

10.06—8. In a patient with generalized bone disease and the following findings in blood chemistry and bone biopsy, what diagnosis is suggested?

10.06. High calcium, low phosphate in blood: numerous osteoclasts in bone	A. Achondroplasia B. Hyperparathyroidism C. Paget's disease
10.07. Low normal calcium, low phosphate: wide osteoid seams	D. Multiple myeloma E. Rickets.
10.08. Normal calcium and phosphate, high alkaline phosphatase: mosaic pattern.	

Answers overleaf

10.04. U.

Once bone is calcified, the calcified tissue can only be removed by osteoclasts. R does not occur naturally.

10.05. Z.

The vast majority of secondaries occur in trunk bones, and the proximal ends of the limbs, and the skull: probably because red marrow areas have the higher blood flow. V refers to "osteoclastic" and "osteoplastic" forms: W to the "leucoerythroblastic anaemia" resulting from displacement of red marrow from its normal site.

10.06. B.

Primary, of course, i.e. due to a parathyroid adenoma: in the secondary variety (e.g. in chronic uraemia) the phosphate is not low.

10.07. E.

Or, of course, osteomalacia if an adult. One would expect the calcium to be low, but is in fact usually only at the lower limits of normal.

10.08. C.

10.09. Generalized bone disease associated with especially **high** incidence of multiple renal stones?

    F. Fragilitas ossium
    G. Hyperparathyroidism
    H. Marble bone disease
    J. Osteoporosis
    K. Paget's disease.

10.10. Tuberculous arthritis affects chiefly?

    L. Fingers
    M. Hip or knee
    N. Sterno-clavicular
    O. Temporomandibular
    P. Wrist or ankle.

10.11. _NOT_ a probable cause of atrophy of calf muscles?

    Q. Amputation of foot at ankle
    R. Blockage of posterior tibial artery at mid-calf level
    S. Division of sciatic nerve
    T. Poliomyelitis
    U. Prolonged confinement to bed.

(e) 10.12. Incidence of metastases of malignant tumour in the voluntary muscles?

    V. One of the commonest sites
    W. Moderately common
    X. Average
    Y. Much less common than might be expected from their size and vascularity
    Z. Nil.

Answers overleaf

10.09. G.

More cases are now diagnosed from investigation of stones than from investigation of bone disease, and in fact many patients (perhaps those who have a high calcium intake in their diet) have stones but no detectable bone lesions. Paget's disease has a doubtful small increase of stones, and any of these diseases *might* have them as a result of the patient's being bedridden.

10.10. M.

Probably chiefly because they are the biggest joints. A fairly safe guess for most bacterial infections, though gonococcal goes for wrist and ankle often.

10.11. R.

This is much too low down to produce ischaemic atrophy in the calf, especially as the anterior tibial and peroneal are available. Q and U cause disuse atrophy, S and T neural atrophy.

10.12. Y.

Reason for this quite unknown. Size for size, even less common than in the spleen. You could not be greatly blamed for answering Z, but absolutes like this are rare in medicine. (See Appendix.)

10.13. A patient whose muscles appear to act normally at first but to tire easily, so that for instance he (or more often she) can open the eyes normally on waking but finds it harder and harder to lift the upper lids as the day goes on, has probably a muscular disease associated with which endocrine organ?

    A. Adrenal medulla
    B. Pineal
    C. Posterior pituitary
    D. Thymus
    E. Thyroid.

10.14—17. Characteristic of osteosarcoma:

    10.14. Arises mainly from the flat bones and vertebrae T/F?
    10.15. Highly radiosensitive and prognosis relatively good T/F?

(e)   10.16. Peak incidence between 5 and 20 years T/F?
    10.17. When found in the elderly, usually in bones affected by Paget's disease T/F?

10.18—21. Characteristic of rheumatoid arthritis:

    10.18. Dense lymphocyte and plasma cell infiltrate in synovium T/F?

(e)   10.19. Involvement chiefly of large proximal joints of limbs T/F?
    10.20. Nodules formed subcutaneously over pressure points T/F?
    10.21. Rheumatoid factor demonstrable by Paul-Bunnell reaction T/F?

Answers overleaf

10.13. D.

This is probably myasthenia gravis. The reason for the relation to the thymus is unknown, though it has recently been shown that there are muscle elements in some thymic cells. About 10% have normal thymus, 10% thymic tumours, and 80% follicular hyperplasia.

10.14. F.

Chiefly from the long bones of the limbs, near their ends.

10.15. F.

Radiosensitivity and prognosis poor (about 20% 5 year survival at best).

10.16. T.

10.17. T.

Very uncommon in elderly in absence of Paget's disease.

10.18. T.

10.19. F.

Peripheral joints most often and characteristically involved — hand and foot, wrist and ankle especially: though *any* joint can be involved.

10.20. T.

Both these and the synovial changes can be of use for diagnosis by biopsy.

10.21. F.

Rose-Waaler, not Paul-Bunnell (which relates to infectious mononucleosis) though both use sheep red cells.

Nervous

(e) 10.22. What lesion of the brain is especially associated with multiple fractures elsewhere in the body?

    F. Contrecoup
    G. Fat embolism
    H. Middle meningeal haemorrhage
    J. Subarachnoid haemorrhage
    K. Thrombosis of longitudinal sinus.

10.23. <u>NOT</u> usually a site of demyelinization?

    L. Plaques of disseminated sclerosis
    M. Posterior column of cord above a lesion involving it
    N. Post-vaccinial encephalitis lesions
    O. Pyramidal tract below an old internal capsule lesion
    P. Sacral plexus cords above a mid-thigh sciatic nerve transection.

10.24–26. Most probable diagnosis (from those given) with these CSF findings (all have high protein).

    10.24. High pressure, very faintly opalescent, many lymphocytes, sugar normal

(e)   10.25. High pressure, turbid, very many polymorphs, sugar absent

    10.26. Low pressure, yellowish and opalescent, few cells, sugar normal.

    Q. Disseminated sclerosis
    R. Pneumococcal meningitis
    S. Viral meningitis
    T. Subarachnoid haemorrhage
    U. Total spinal block.

(e) 10.27. In polio (acute anterior poliomyelitis) the essential early lesion is?

    V. Anaphylactic damage to motor nerve end plates
    W. Death of anterior horn cells with polymorph infiltration
    X. Pressure atrophy of pyramidal tracts
    Y. Viral infection of anterior nerve roots
    Z. Viral myositis.

Answers overleaf

10.22. G.

An important cause of death in major trauma. F and H, and J as well (though not in its usual form), are associated with fractures of the skull itself.

10.23. P.

Demyelinization of a peripheral nerve only extends proximally as far as the next node of Ranvier. M and O are tract degenerations on the side away from the neurone: L and N are demyelinating diseases.

10.24. S.

One would of course also have to think of tuberculous meningitis, especially if working in an area where this is still common: but in that case spider web clot, low chloride and demonstration of the tubercle bacillus will usually distinguish the case from the otherwise often similar findings in virus meningitis.

10.25. R.

Simply a watery purulent exudate.

10.26. U.

This is Froin's syndrome, due to locking up a pool of CSF from its normal circulation.

10.27. W.

A highly specific localization of the virus to anterior horn cells.

10.28. Middle-meningeal haemorrhage has a characteristic history of brief unconsciousness after a blow on the head, rapid return to normal, and then relapse into coma after some hours. What is happening during the lucid interval?

    A. Bleeding between dura and arachnoid
    B. Formation of haematoma between skull and dura
    C. Increasing hydrocephalus
    D. Spreading thrombosis of middle meningeal, ultimately involving carotid
    E. Spreading thrombosis of neighbouring venous sinuses.

(e) 10.29. The commonest site of an "ordinary" cerebral haemorrhage is?

    F. Basal ganglia
    G. Cerebellum
    H. Corpus callosum
    J. Pons
    K. Temporal lobe

10.30.—32. Probable cause of extensive necrosis in the brain with the distribution suggested?

10.30. Basal ganglia and all tissues round the lateral sulcus on one side	L. Herpes simplex encephalitis
10.31. Boundary zones between territories of main cerebral arteries	M. Longitudinal venous sinus thrombosis
10.32. Cortical grey matter of most of cerebrum, worst over temporal lobes.	N. Middle cerebral artery block
	O. Posterior cerebellar artery block
	P. Prolonged low blood pressure or anoxia.

10.28. B.

This is where the artery lies, extradurally, and the tough attachment of dura to bone means bleeding is slow, and hence the build-up to a size at which it compresses and distorts the brain is slow. Arterial bleeding anywhere else in the cranium is usually a rapid affair.

10.29. F.

G and J are the only other reasonably common sites.

10.30. N.

The classical thrombotic stroke.

10.31. P.

When blood is poor in quantity or quality, the areas farthest from the main trunk are most affected.

10.32. L.

Severe herpes encephalitis produces exceptionally severe and extensive damage to grey matter. This is one of the conditions in which often the quickest way of making a diagnosis is by electron microscopy on a biopsy.

(e) **10.33.** <u>NOT</u> **produced by an expanding lesion within the right cerebral hemisphere?**

    Q. Compression of right lateral ventricle
    R. Displacement of third ventricle to right
    S. Flattening of convolutions
    T. Herniations of brain tissue under falx and tentorium
    U. Raised intra-cranial pressure.

10.34. Particularly likely to cause hydrocephalus involving the third and both lateral ventricles but not the fourth?

    V. Astrocytoma of cerebellum
    W. Excessive production of CSF
    X. Glioblastoma of frontal lobe
    Y. Meningioma over occipital lobe
    Z. Tuberculous meningitis.

(e) **10.35. Cell type that gives rise to the largest group of primary tumours of the central nervous system?**

    A. Endothelium of vessels
    B. Meninges
    C. Mesoglia
    D. Nerve cells
    E. Neuroglia.

10.36. The neuroblastoma, one of the commonest malignant tumours of children, in spite of its name arises not in the brain but most often in the?

    F. Adrenal medulla
    G. Anterior nerve roots of spinal cord
    H. Filum terminale
    J. Ganglia of vagus nerve
    K. Peripheral nerves.

Answers overleaf

10.33. R.

The third ventricle, with all the other mid-line structures, is pushed *away* from the tumour. This is the kind of over-obvious answer that people often miss just because it is below the level of difficulty they expect in the question. Though a good paper will avoid them as far as possible, here this at least tests remembrance of elementary anatomy.

10.34. V.

This will compress the fourth ventricle and prevent flow of CSF out of the other three. Of the others only Z is especially likely to produce hydrocephalus, and since the block here is in the foramina giving exit from the fourth ventricle the latter is also dilated. W *can* produce some hydrocephalus, but again involving all ventricles, and only as a great rarity resulting from an actively secreting tumour of the choroid plexus.

10.35. E.

This is the origin of the gliomas, which include ependymomas and oligodendrogliomas as well as the astrocytomas.

10.36. F.

It arises usually from the adrenal medulla, but also from sympathetic ganglia: remember their common origin and the similar distribution of phaeochromocytoma. Its newer name of sympathicoblastoma indicates this origin.

10.37—41. Often accompanied by peripheral neuropathy:

    10.37. Carcinoma of bronchus T/F?
    10.38. Herpes zoster T/F?
    10.39. Lead poisoning T/F?
    10.40. Vit. B_1 deficiency T/F?
    10.41. Diabetes mellitus T/F?

Skin

10.42—45. True of malignant melanoma:

    10.42. Presence of melanin essential to the diagnosis T/F?
    10.43. Proportion of benign pigmented naevi that give rise to malignant melanomas is minute T/F?
    10.44. Skin is the only important site of origin T/F?
    10.45. Very rare before puberty T/F?

Answers overleaf

10.37. T.

10.38. F.

The lesion being in the posterior root ganglion, which is not part of the peripheral nerve according to the anatomists.

10.39. T.

Painter's colic is or was often accompanied by dropped wrist.

10.40. T.

"Dry beri-beri".

10.41. T.

(All of these are in one way or another associated with a CNS disease — some rather recondite, but do you know any of them? See Deferred Notes.)

10.42. F.

Totally amelanotic melanomas are not rare, and even in the usual type it may be patchy.

10.43. T.

Do not confuse this with its converse — many malignant melanomata arise in naevi (one third to one half) but naevi are much commoner than melanomas.

10.44. F.

Apart from rare sites like nose, rectum and meninges, it is the commonest malignant tumour of the eye.

10.45. T.

10.46. <u>NOT</u> a site specially liable to squamous carcinoma of the skin?

    L. Back of hand of fair-skinned outdoor workers
    M. Face of fair-skinned in sunny climates
    N. Face of sufferers from xeroderma pigmentosa
    O. Edges of long-standing ulcers and sinuses
    P. Shoulders of coal-heavers.

Answers overleaf

10.46. P.

At least no association seems to have been recorded and in general coal dust is not carcinogenic.

M. applies much more to rodent ulcers, but squamous carcinoma is also significantly increased in incidence. This is the kind of question one can quite legitimately answer by exclusion.

11. REVISION

A few questions of a different type for general revision, with an emphasis on cause and effect. They consist of two statements separated by the word BECAUSE, the second purporting to be the cause of the first. Answer them as follows:

A. Both statements true, and the second acceptable as a cause of the first
B. Both statements true, but not causally related
C. First statement true, second false
D. First statement false, second true
E. Both false.

11.01. In acute inflammation very little reabsorption of exudate occurs at the venous end of the capillaries BECAUSE increased capillary permeability leads to loss of the osmotic pressure gradient normally present at this point.

11.02. Complete resolution of catarrhal inflammation is unusual BECAUSE this kind of inflammation involves destruction of underlying connective tissue as well as epithelium.

11.03. Adhesions are often a consequence of acute inflammation of a serous membrane BECAUSE the fibrinous exudate which forms between the opposed surfaces is especially liable to undergo organization.

Answers overleaf

11.01. A.

The permeability acts in two ways: (a) because the capillary wall is no longer an efficient semipermeable membrane and (b) because proteins already leaked out reduce the osmotic pressure difference.

11.02. E.

Neither is true. Catarrhal inflammation practically always resolves (e.g. common cold): the second half describes pseudo-membranous (diphtheritic) inflammation.

11.03. A.

This is the classical mode of formation of adhesions, e.g. in peritoneum.

11.04. When both circulating antibodies and sensitized lymphocytes are present which can each separately react with injected cells (e.g. of a transplantable tumour) the lymphocytes are often prevented from acting to destroy the injected cells BECAUSE the antibody reacts with the receptors on the surface of the lymphocyte.

11.05. In the form of congenital immunological deficiency in which the primary defect is in the thymus, skin grafts from donors survive better than usual BECAUSE rejection of such grafts depends on a cellular immune reaction.

11.06. The proportion of the people who die of cancer in most under-developed societies is very much lower than in western Europe BECAUSE their exposure to industrial carcinogens is much less.

11.07. Haemosiderin is deposited in the liver in most cases of anaemia (excepting iron-deficiency anaemia) BECAUSE when the marrow is hyperactive for any cause there is usually increased absorption of iron from the intestine.

11.08. Infarcts are much more often caused by thrombosis of arteries than of veins (even though thrombosis of veins is commoner) BECAUSE end-arteries are much commoner than end-veins.

Answers overleaf

11.04. C.

The antibody reacts with and blocks the antigen on the surface of the injected cells, not with the lymphocytes.

11.05. A.

The homograft (or allograft) reaction depends on a cellular response: grafts protected from sensitized lymphocytes (e.g. on the cornea) survive indefinitely.

This is the Di George syndrome, in which parathyroids are also deficient. Fungal and virus infections are commonest. In the gamma globulin deficiencies, it is pyogenic bacteria that cause most trouble.

11.06. B.

The bulk of the difference depends on age at death: except for very heavy exposure to active carcinogens, the cancer death rate depends chiefly on the number of people who survive into the decades over 50 when cancer becomes common.

11.07. B.

Both facts are true, and the second fact gives rise to heavy iron overload in some cases of very longstanding marrow activity (e.g. thalassaemia), but the usual reason for the iron excess in the liver in, for instance, P.A. and aplastic anaemia, is that the red cell mass is reduced and the iron in the missing red cells has to be stored somewhere.

11.08. A.

The rarity of end-veins probably is a defence against their much greater tendency to blockage, either by thrombosis or pressure. Where a single vein serves an organ, as with kidney or especially the adrenal, venous blockage does cause infarction. Of course emboli also weight the incidence towards arteries, but this question refers to thrombosis, by which one assumes a local process.

11.09. Rupture of a myocardial infarct is most likely to occur about 25 days after its formation BECAUSE at that time the infarct is softest and weakest.

11.10. Farmer's lung is essentially an alveolitis BECAUSE inhaled antigen combines with circulating antibody in the alveolar wall.

11.11. Cancer of the stomach has a much worse prognosis than cancer of the colon BECAUSE it has a much greater effect on nutrition.

11.12. Banting and Best, who discovered insulin, were unable to extract it from the pancreas until they used glands whose duct had been tied some weeks earlier BECAUSE blocked-duct atrophy eliminates the trypsin-secreting tissue and spares the islets.

11.13. If a patient with obstructive jaundice has a distended gall bladder, the cause is more likely to be a stone in the common bile duct than carcinoma of the pancreas BECAUSE in the latter condition the gall bladder is likely to be chronically inflamed and will therefore distend more easily.

11.14. In haemolytic anaemia the urine remains light in colour BECAUSE the bilirubin in the blood is conjugated and so cannot pass through the glomerular filter.

Answers overleaf

11.09. E.

Both are wrong. But substitute 10 days for 25 and the answer is A. At ten days autolysis is maximum, but after that time formation of collagen strengthens the area. But rupture can occur at almost any time, from about 2nd day till years later: in the late ones the fibrous area usually undergoes aneurysmal dilatation first.

11.10. A.

Farmer's lung depends on the slow formation of precipitating antibodies in normal individuals as a result of prolonged exposure to large doses of fungal spores and the point where these meet in largest quantity to produce an Arthus reaction is obviously the alveolar wall.

11.11. B.

It does produce malnutrition more rapidly, but its higher death rate is due chiefly to its much poorer differentiation and more rapid dissemination than is the case with the colon.

11.12. A.

So the trypsin could not hydrolyse the insulin during extraction. Actually in time the islets atrophy also.

11.13. E.

This is a travesty of the truth. Courvoisier's law (which works out fairly well in practice) states that a distended G.B. in a patient with obstructive jaundice indicates carcinoma, and this is because with gall stones the G.B. is usually fibrosed and so unable to distend.

11.14. C.

It is because the bilirubin is *not* conjugated that it cannot pass into the urine: conjugation makes it water-soluble and hence filtrable.

11.15. In those inborn errors of metabolism in which the thyroid is unable to concentrate iodine, the level of TSH is depressed BECAUSE the enlarged thyroid produces more thyroxin than normal.

11.16. Cancer of the uterine cervix often produces uraemia terminally BECAUSE lymph spread produces para-aortic secondaries round the renal vessels.

11.17. If one crosses a strain of mice with a high incidence of breast cancer with a low-cancer strain, the incidence of breast cancer in the offspring depends usually entirely on the father and not at all on the mother BECAUSE the Bittner factor is transmitted in the milk.

11.18. In sickle cell anaemia, the heterozygotes suffer from the disease BECAUSE their red cells contain Haemoglobin S.

11.19. In multiple myelomatosis the γ-globulin in the blood forms a high narrow spike on the electrophoresis tracing BECAUSE myelocytes can produce γ-globulin only of this one particular variety.

11.20. Inadequate or delayed treatment of acute bacterial meningitis may save life but leave a sequel of hydro-cephalus BECAUSE the foramina in the roof of the fourth ventricle become blocked.

Answers overleaf

11.15. E.

Both are false, though of course *if* the thyroid produced excessive thyroxin TSH would be depressed. In fact if the thyroid cannot trap iodine thyroxin production is reduced, and the pituitary feed-back ensures that TSH rises — hence the thyroid enlargement.

11.16. B.

Though both statements are true, para-aortic tumour deposits rarely seem to block the renal vessels. Uraemia in these cases is usually due to direct invasion of the ureters where they run forward beside the two vaginal lateral fornices.

11.17. D.

It is of course the *mother* who determines the incidence. The Bittner virus is transmitted in the milk and produces cancer in female offspring late in their life.

11.18. D.

They do not suffer from the disease, although their red cells contain the abnormal haemoglobin, because the normal gene on the other chromosome produces enough normal haemoglobin to prevent trouble in the red cells except when conditions are extreme, as in the laboratory sickling test. Heterozygotes are said to show the sickle-cell *trait*.

11.19. C.

The cells in myelomatosis are plasma cells (of one clone, hence producing only one kind of γ-globulin in any one case), not myelocytes, which are polymorph precursors and do not produce γ-globulin. The type of globulin differs from case to case.

11.20. A.

The inflammatory exudate in meningitis behaves like any other if it is allowed to persist, and the organization which then occurs has as its most dangerous consequence the blockage of the CSF outlet around the medulla.

12. DEFERRED NOTES

These are the answers to various subsidiary questions which it seemed possible you might have been moved to ask after reading the answers to some of the original questions.

1.02.

Some kind of marrow damage leading to defective production of neutrophiles — effect of radiation or drugs, leukaemia, or the unexplained failure of neutrophile production called "idiopathic agranulocytosis". Overwhelming infection can sometimes prevent leucocytosis. And of course there are many infections (most non-bacterial, but including typhoid) in which leucopenia is usual.

1.09.

Covering a wound surface with epidermis in this way is valuable, for it protects the raw surface. But if it grows over granulation tissue, the resultant fibrous tissue will in time reduce its volume and produce the effect of a contracted scar. Only surviving dermis (which does not regenerate) can prevent this.

2.08.

Reasonable guesses might be: M, coliforms; N, pneumococci or pyocyaneus; O, amoebiasis ("anchovy sauce" in hepatic abscess); P, *Streptococcus pyogenes*.

2.09. (a)

Opportunistic infection occurs with organisms of low virulence when the immunity of the host is abnormally depressed.

2.09. (b)

R is the protozoon that causes the commonest form of malaria.
S is an itch mite (an arachnid) that causes scabies. T is a tape-
worm that causes hydatid disease, mostly in sheep-rearing areas.
U is the protozoon of toxoplasmosis, a very common infection
in mild form that can cause major damage in babies.

3.07.

Krukenberg tumour. Spread of cancer cells (usually gastric)
via the peritoneum into the ovary (before the menopause)
produces a very peculiar massive fibrous tumour of the ovary.

3.08.

Yes, probably at least. Breast carcinoma secondaries in the
vertebral bodies are commonest in the mid-thoracic area, and
nasopharyngeal carcinoma in the upper cervical area, and are
probably vein-spread.

3.11.

Erythropoietin. Renin secretion is very rare, and the tumours
which secrete it are benign and of a very specialized type, their
cells resembling those of the juxta-glomerular apparatus.

4.12—4.14.

Morgagni, an eighteenth century Italian, wrote the first text-
book of pathology ('Of the seats and causes of diseases').
Aschoff was the top German pathologist of the inter-war years
and described "Aschoff's nodes" in the heart in acute
rheumatism. (Noone will fail you for not knowing the history
of pathology: but it prejudices examiners in your favour if you
can occasionally show some evidence of interest in the back-
ground of medicine.)

5.03.

Effects are L. Cerebral infarct ("softening") which is often fatal. M. Sudden death (from massive pulmonary embolism). N. Myocardial infarct. P. Infarct of gut ("mesenteric thrombosis").

5.10.

Children around the age of five. The great majority of other causes of death are at their lowest between 5 and 15.

5.15.

Large vegetations would mean bacterial endocarditis, occurring *after* the mitral stenosis (hence M, P, L, O, N). Pin head vegetations would be acute rheumatic, part of the original rheumatic fever attack.

5.29—5.33.

With free communication between the ventricles, the pressure in both must be nearly equal. On the right it then must be abnormally high, and hence

5.29. Hypertrophy.

5.30. PA pressure is hence also high, from birth, so its wall is thick.

5.31. The pressure is still higher on the left, hence flow is left to right, not the reverse.

5.32. Hence no venous blood reaches the L.V., and there is no cyanosis. (If the pulmonary artery pressure rises, flow may be reversed and cyanosis appear, but this usually brings signs of heart failure; and it is not the usual state of an uncomplicated septal defect).

5.33. Most congenital heart lesions carry a risk of SABE, especially those that cause abnormalities of flow of L.V. blood.

6.07.

F. Tuberculous bronchopneumonia is usually a terminal lesion, either in child or adult. G. Part of the primary complex, nearly always in childhood. J. Result of healing: usually chiefly towards apex. K. Often accompanies the early stages of a mild attack in a young adult — used to be common in medical students.

7.03.

Most of the squamous epithelium of the pharynx is closely associated with lymphoid tissue of the tonsil-adenoid ring, and tumours of this area seem usually to involve lymphoid aggregates. But the epithelium is the neoplastic element. Carcinoma of the pharynx has two odd epidemiological features: a specially high incidence in Chinese, and an association with the EB virus similar to that of Burkitt's tumour.

7.08.

A, fibrous stricture, is only important in duodenal ulcers, though it also sometimes occurs with oesophageal ulcers. Hour-glass stricture of the mid-stomach, once common in women, seem to have practically vanished. D, malignancy, does not occur in the duodenum.

7.14.

He presumably has extensive atheroma and 'thrombophilia'. He may have independent thrombi in femoral and superior mesenteric arteries, but he may rather more probably have a massive thrombus developing in the lower aorta, involving iliacs at one end and mesenteric at the other. An atheromatous aneurysm of the lower part of the aorta is also possible, but this will also produce its effects by the thrombosis in and near it.

7.22.

M. Kala-azar. N. Malaria (benign tertian form). O. Toxo-plasmosis. P. Sleeping sickness.

7.35.

Q. Prostatic carcinoma. R. Obstructive jaundice and bone diseases. T. Muscular dystrophy (and cardiac infarcts). U. Liver damage and cardiac infarcts.

8.03.

The nephrotic syndrome can be produced by any form of glomerulonephritis with long-continued albuminuria (subacute progressive, membranous, minimum-change) and by a variety of other conditions — amyloidosis and Kimmelstiel-Wilson (diabetic kidney) are enough to remember at this stage. Remember that oedema due to low serum albumen can have other causes — starvation (kwashiorkor) and protein leak from the gut.

8.06.

R. Diabetes mellitus. S. Nephrotic syndrome. T. Dehydration. U. Acute infections of the urinary tract.

8.49.

M. Laennec (macronodular) and Hanot (primary biliary). N. Hodgkin. O. Bright. P. von Recklinghausen. The last of these also described hyperparathyroidism. Addison (disease and anaemia) and Pott (fracture and spine) also have important double eponyms, and among rarer diseases there are many more.

9.35.

Transfusion. If it was enough to bring the haemoglobin back to normal, there would be little stimulus to excessive new blood formation.

9.36.

She must be a carrier, a fact made more obvious by the link with the maternal uncle. Since she is not clinically affected, she must have only one X chromosome involved: the other is normal and produces enough AHG to prevent disease. So she is a heterozygous carrier of an abnormal gene on one of her X chromosomes.

10.37—10.41.

10.37. Cerebellar ataxia (very rare).

10.38. Rather remote, but varicella (caused by the same virus) is sometimes followed by post-infectious (demyelinating) encephalitis.

10.39. Lead encephalopathy.

10.40. Cerebral beri-beri (Wernicke's encephalopathy).

10.41. Cerebral thrombosis due to atheroma — another rather indirect connexion.

APPENDIX:
SOME ADVICE ON ANSWERING
M.C.Q. PAPERS

My only experience as a candidate since qualifying has been an army examination in elementary Malay in 1941 and a very friendly Ph.D. viva in 1953, and I have never sat an M.C.Q. paper in earnest in my life, so this attempt to offer advice might seem to resemble that of a cat advising mice how to avoid being eaten. But one would hope that most undergraduates by the time they reach pathology are capable of regarding examinations as at the worst a necessary evil. Failure is a necessary warning that one is not pulling one's weight: success a strong support to the morale, a confirmation that one is not after all as inadequate and incompetent as one sometimes imagined. But before the candidate can accept this view, he must be confident that the examination is as efficient as possible and administered with ruthless fairness. These are matters for the examiners: but also he must be confident that he will not suffer from inadequate understanding of the method of examining.

M.C.Q. form within their limitations the most efficient simple method of examination available in most subjects. They derive their efficiency from two things: (a) a short paper can cover a very wide field, so that patchy knowledge is adequately sampled and (b) there is no possible ambiguity about the marks given for each paper. Obviously they test factual knowledge best, and there are many necessary aspects of medical skill where they are of little use (at least without great complications) so that most examinations need to use a variety of techniques. Nevertheless it is worth being certain that you understand the way M.C.Q. work well enough to make sure that you do not lose marks to which you are entitled by the standard of your knowledge of the subject.

Marking systems

Before settling down to practical advice, it is as well to make sure you understand marking. While some very elaborate systems

145

have been proposed (weighting wrong answers for different
degrees of wrongness, for instance, or allowing candidates to vary
their stakes by indicating different degrees of confidence in their
choices), in practice you can expect that in all cases you will
receive one mark for each correct answer, and to receive a
constant minus mark, a *countermark*, for each wrong answer.

The no penalty system. The countermark may be 0, your score
being made up of the total of correct choices with no notice
being taken of wrong choices. This is a common practice in the
U.S., in elementary schools, and in intelligence tests, but unusual
in senior examinations in this country. In case you encounter it,
however, you must understand its effect. There is no penalty for
guessing at all. (The examiner of course has no way of telling
whether you guessed or not). So with this system you *must*
answer *every* question. Since chance will always give you some
right answers, even when you know nothing, you will lose marks
in comparison with those who guess if you leave any question
unanswered. On this system, chance will average 50% on 100 TF
questions, or 20% on one-from-fives.

The "fair" countermark. This is the system you are most likely
to encounter in this country. Here the countermark is set at such
a level that guessing will on average produce neither loss or gain.
For a one-from-five this is $-1/4$, and for a TF it is -1. Random
guessing you will find produces an average score of nil in both
cases. So while with no countermark you *must* guess every time,
here you can choose whether to guess or not.

There are two aspects of this worth considering, however.
First, if you know enough to be able to eliminate some of the
answers in a one-from-five, it is always worth guessing among
the last two or three, for the odds are in your favour. Second,
you should realise that, just as tossing ten coins on *average* will
produce five heads, but will often turn up two or eight and even
rarely nought or ten, the score you make on guesses will vary a
good deal from that expected. So in the "fair" system you have
an even chance of gaining or losing by guessing. It follows from
this that if you are reasonably sure that you have reached a pass
mark without blind guessing, you should avoid risking any but

the best bets, for otherwise guessing badly may bring you
down below the fail mark.

Heavier countermarking. Since guessing, because of the chance
element, reduces the accuracy of the final mark, there is a
good deal to be said for a countermark that penalizes the wilder
degrees of guessing. It is however still unusual, and you will be
warned if the countermark is, say, $-1/3$. Of course, since countermarks affect the final scores, adjustments have to be made
either to the difficulty of questions or the pass mark. If you do
not like heavy countermarks, consider Will Rogers' saying:
"The trouble isn't what people don't know: it's what they do
know that isn't so".

Relative values of questions. It requires more thought to pick a
right answer out of five than out of two, so a one-from-five is
worth more than a TF. This is of no great importance to the
candidate, and mentioned here only to explain the different
marks suggested for the two kinds in the introduction. The fact
that the best ratio is disputed is one good reason for not mixing
the two in one examination.

Multiple answering. A small point is the method of dealing with
cases where a candidate has marked more than one of the
possible answers to a question. It is usual and simplest, and on
the whole I think best, to treat all such as one wrong answer.
Sometimes however the two are marked separately, so that if
one of them is right the result is 1 mark for the right one and
$-1/4$ for the other, i.e. $3/4$ in all. If that is the case you ought to
be told about it, for one could then make multiple answers as a
deliberate policy if for instance one was sure that the correct
answer was one of two.

Practical management

Read the instructions. If there is a front sheet telling you what
to do, or a notice on the door, *read it.* Even if you have done it
all before, the examiners may have changed the rules without
telling you, or announced it at a lecture you missed — incon-
siderate but, if it is in the instructions, legal. Make sure you
know and understand the rules of *this* particular examination.
If in doubt, ask the invigilator: it is one of the things he is there
for.

Timing. You should by now have learnt to pace yourself in examinations. You *must* get right through the M.C.Q. paper in the time available. In an essay paper it is sometimes profitable to go all out on the subject you know and hope that a kindly examiner will believe that only shortness of time curtailed your answers to the rest: but quantity overall is what counts in M.C.Q. You get marks for correct answers, none for sitting thinking about them, and it is no use wasting time scratching for marks in the middle when there may be gold on the last page. Work out roughly the time you have per question (probably something between 30 seconds and a minute). There is no problem with the easiest or the hardest questions, where you recognize at once whether you know or do not know the answer. For the grey ones which need thinking about, unless you are ahead of schedule, make a note of them and leave them. Then you should be able to reach the end with time in hand to think about the harder ones you have left behind, without risking missing any easy questions.

Guessing. Policy on this should be obvious if you know the mark scheme and have read the previous section. In general, with the usual "fair" system, it is unwise to be too inhibited about guessing. If you believe the chances of being right are substantially better than the blind odds recognized by the countermark (e.g. if you can eliminate two, or, better, three of the five possible answers) guessing ought to show a profit. But do not guess entirely blindly.

Miscellaneous points chiefly applicable to one-from-fives

(a) It is fatally easy to miss *negatives* in the question. Not all examiners are obliging enough to make their <u>*NOT*</u>'s as conspicuous as they are in this book.

(b) There is nothing wrong about exclusion as a method of finding the right answer. "Tumour of lymph nodes in children? A. Amyloid, B. Cirrhosis, C. Fibroma, D. Letterer-Siwe disease, E. Smallpox". You may never have heard of Letterer-Siwe, but since none of the others can be right, it is at the very least worth trying.

(c) Examiners sometimes, either through inexperience or carelessness, drop broad hints to the wideawake — a plural verb in the question and only one plural answer, say, or a question asking for the name of a part of the body when some of the answers are names of diseases. Incompatible questions dragged into the group format are particularly liable to this. Do not scruple to take advantage of these lapses but (not in any pull-the-ladder-up spirit, but in the interest of good examining, which we are agreed is for the good of both parties) see he is told about it afterwards.

(d) In grouped one-from-fives it is usually safe to assume that an answer used once can be eliminated from the remaining questions in the group. Some examiners, with good reason, are prepared to use answers more than once, but in view of the usual practice, ought to warn you that they are doing so.

Points related chiefly to true-falses

(a) The usual regular lay-out of these in sets of five can make them look very like one-from-fives: be quite certain you do not confuse them.

(b) Absolutes are rare in medicine. "Never" and "always" and "exactly 7.222" usually signal a false statement. But this rule is itself dangerously near to an absolute. "Pure XO Turner's syndrome female are always infertile" is still true I believe if you strictly define the syndrome: and severed long C.N.S. tracts never return to normal: but such examples are not numerous.

(c) If the TF's are grouped as usual in fives, most examiners are unwilling to make all five right or all five wrong. There is no reason why they should not, and you might well be justified in inquiring as to local practice in this matter.

Other question types. This book covers all the question types in general use in this country, though there are of course many minor variants in format. Most techniques of examination by computer or other mechanized devices are basically M.C.Q. variants, though of course complications are frequent.

Off-beat question types are chiefly troublesome because of the effort of bending one's mind to a new technique in the middle of an examination. The BECAUSE questions of Chapter XI are included chiefly for this reason. An easy example of one other style is given here, solely to ensure that if you ever meet it you will not have to spend too long wondering how it works.

Appendix

Choose one item from each of the following two lists, such that all the other four items in the first list produce or cause the chosen one in the second list.

A.	Aplasia of marrow	X.	Anaemia
B.	Cancer of stomach	Y.	Peritonitis
C.	Deficiency of folic acid	Z.	Swelling of lower
D.	Duodenal ulcer		abdomen.
E.	Simple cyst of ovary		

(Answer E, X)

Finally

M.C.Q. appear to be with us to stay, and with the increase of postgraduate examinations you can expect to continue to be faced with them to an advanced age. If you still find them troublesome, here are two suggestions:

(a) Persuade your teachers to spend an occasional small-group session on a recent paper, and use some of it to discuss why the right answers are right.

(b) Make up a few questions of your own, and try them on your friends. You will soon increase your understanding of the process.

Remember no examination is absolutely accurate — even M.C.Q. You must allow at the least 5% for error. If you allow less, and by bad luck fail, blame only your own bad judgement.

Remember again that an accurate assessment is for your good and your fellow students' good: and, while it is a pity to fail through lack of examination technique, anything that gives anyone a better mark than he deserves, or favours one group of students at the expense of another, is in the long run equally undesirable to all concerned.